Medicaid & Medicare

-

The Comprehensive Guide

by

VIRUTI SHIVAN

Masters in Clinical Psychology (Major)

"In books, as in life, it's not the size or looks but

the content that matters."

Introduction

Welcome to "Medicaid & Medicare - The Comprehensive Guide," a journey through the labyrinth of the United States' major health care programs. If you've ever found yourself puzzled by the intricacies of Medicaid and Medicare, you're not alone. These programs, vital to millions, can often seem like a complex puzzle with constantly shifting pieces. But fear not! This guide is here to turn confusion into clarity, questions into answers.

Imagine Medicaid and Medicare as two distinct characters in the vast narrative of the U.S. healthcare system. Medicaid, with its state-level nuances and income-based eligibility, is like a chameleon, constantly adapting to the environment of each state's policies and demographics. Medicare, on the other hand, is the steady, reliable tortoise, moving at a consistent pace, providing healthcare support mainly to those over 65, regardless of income.

Throughout this book, we'll embark on a storytelling adventure, weaving through the history, structures, and essential details of these programs. We'll debunk myths, unveil hidden truths, and provide practical tips and exercises to help you navigate these waters with confidence.

But why is understanding these programs so crucial, you ask? Simply put, knowledge is power. Whether you're a beneficiary, a caregiver, a healthcare professional, or just planning ahead, knowing the ins and outs of Medicaid and Medicare can have a profound impact on your health, finances, and peace of mind.

So, let's turn the page and begin this enlightening journey together. By the end of this guide, you'll not only have a thorough understanding of Medicaid and Medicare but also the tools and knowledge to make informed decisions about your healthcare future. Welcome aboard!

Chapter 1: Understanding the Basics of Medicaid and Medicare

1.1. Overview of Medicaid

Dive into the world of Medicaid, a key player in the U.S. health care system designed to assist those in need. Picture Medicaid as a safety net, elegantly woven with threads of federal and state policies, stretching out to catch individuals and families who might otherwise fall through the cracks of the healthcare system.

Medicaid: The Basics

At its core, Medicaid is a joint venture between the federal government and individual states. Each state tailors its Medicaid program within federal guidelines, which is why Medicaid can look quite different from one state to another. Think of it as a chameleon, changing colors depending on its environment. The program primarily serves low-income individuals, families, pregnant women, the elderly, and people with disabilities.

Who Qualifies?

Eligibility for Medicaid is like a puzzle with pieces that include income, family size, and special circumstances. Generally, if your income falls below a certain threshold, Medicaid opens its doors to you. However, it's not just about how much you make. Other factors, like age, pregnancy, and disability status, also play a role in determining your eligibility.

Services Covered

Imagine a buffet of healthcare services; that's what Medicaid offers to its beneficiaries. From hospital visits to long-term care, from prenatal services to prescription drugs, the range is broad. Some services are mandatory across all states, like inpatient and outpatient hospital services, while others, like dental coverage for adults, vary by state.

The State-Federal Tango

Picture a dance between the states and the federal government. The federal government sets the basic rhythm with broad requirements and funding, while states add their own unique steps by determining specific eligibility criteria and additional services. This dance results in a diverse array of Medicaid programs across the country, each with its own flavor.

Impact on Lives

Medicaid isn't just a program; it's a lifeline for millions. It provides much-needed medical coverage to the most vulnerable populations, reducing the number of uninsured Americans and improving access to essential healthcare services. For many,

Medicaid is the difference between receiving necessary medical care and facing insurmountable health challenges.

As we journey through the world of Medicaid, keep in mind that it's more than a set of policies and regulations; it's a dynamic entity that adapts and evolves, impacting real lives every day. Whether you're a current or prospective beneficiary, a healthcare provider, or just a curious soul, understanding Medicaid is crucial in comprehending the larger picture of healthcare in the United States.

1.2. Overview of Medicare

Now, let's shift gears to Medicare, the other cornerstone of American healthcare, primarily serving those over 65, regardless of income. If Medicaid is the chameleon of healthcare, then Medicare is its steadfast companion, reliably providing support to a different, but equally important, segment of the population.

Medicare at a Glance

Medicare is a federally run program, a unifying force in the health care mosaic of the United States. It primarily caters to individuals aged 65 and older, but also covers younger people with certain disabilities and those with End-Stage Renal Disease (permanent kidney failure requiring dialysis or a transplant). Picture Medicare as a blanket of security, covering a significant portion of the elder population and others in need.

Understanding the Parts of Medicare

Medicare is like a four-part harmony, each part playing a crucial role:

1. **Part A (Hospital Insurance):** This is the foundation, covering inpatient hospital stays, care in a skilled nursing facility, hospice care, and some home health care. Think of it as your safety net for more significant medical events.

2. **Part B (Medical Insurance):** This covers certain doctors' services, outpatient care, medical supplies, and preventive services. It's like your day-to-day healthcare ally.

3. **Part C (Medicare Advantage Plans):** An alternative to Original Medicare, these are private plans that bundle Part A and B and often include Part D. Imagine a one-stop-shop for all your Medicare needs, sometimes with added benefits.

4. **Part D (Prescription Drug Coverage):** This helps cover the cost of prescription drugs, including many recommended shots or vaccines. Consider this your shield against high medication costs.

Eligibility and Enrollment

Joining Medicare isn't an automatic process for everyone. While some are enrolled automatically at 65, others need to sign up. There are specific enrollment periods, and missing these can mean penalties, so timing is essential. Think of it like catching a train – being on time is crucial.

Coverage and Costs

Medicare isn't a free-for-all. There are premiums, deductibles, and co-pays, much like other insurance plans. However, it often covers a significant portion of healthcare expenses, easing the financial burden that healthcare can pose, especially in retirement years.

The Role of Medicare in Public Health

Medicare does more than just cover medical bills. It's a pillar of public health, ensuring that the aging population has access to necessary medical care. This accessibility is vital for the overall health and well-being of millions of seniors and other eligible individuals, making Medicare a key player in the nation's health.

In summary, Medicare is a comprehensive, federally administered program, a beacon of support for older adults and others who qualify. Understanding its parts, how they work together, and the impact they have is essential for anyone navigating the healthcare landscape, either for themselves or for loved ones.

1.3. Key Differences Between Medicaid and Medicare

Having explored the landscapes of Medicaid and Medicare individually, it's time to put them side by side and examine the key differences. Think of this as a tale of two programs, each with its unique characteristics, yet both integral to the fabric of American healthcare.

Eligibility: Income vs. Age

The most fundamental difference lies in eligibility. Medicaid is primarily designed for low-income individuals and families, with eligibility criteria based on income and other factors like disability and family size. In contrast, Medicare primarily serves people aged 65 and older, regardless of income, as well as younger individuals with certain disabilities and those with End-Stage Renal Disease.

Program Administration: Federal-State Partnership vs. Federal Only

Medicaid is a collaborative dance between the federal government and individual states. Each state runs its own Medicaid program within federal guidelines, leading to variations in coverage and eligibility across the country. Medicare, on the other hand, is a federally administered program, offering a consistent experience nationwide.

Coverage Scope and Services

While there is some overlap in coverage, the scope of services differs between the two. Medicaid often covers a broader range of services, including long-term care, which Medicare typically does not cover. Medicare, divided into Parts A, B, C, and D, focuses on hospital and medical insurance, Medicare Advantage plans, and prescription drug coverage.

Costs to Beneficiaries

The cost structure also varies. Medicaid often has minimal to no costs for covered services for the beneficiaries, thanks to its focus on assisting low-income individuals. Medicare, while subsidizing a significant portion of healthcare costs, usually involves premiums (especially for Part B and D), deductibles, and co-pays.

Flexibility and Portability

Medicaid's state-specific nature means coverage and eligibility can change if you move to a different state. Medicare, being a federal program, offers the same coverage and benefits across the U.S., making it more portable for those who travel or relocate.

Enrollment Periods and Processes

Enrollment processes differ too. Medicaid allows enrollment any time of the year, subject to eligibility. Medicare has specific enrollment periods, and missing these can lead to penalties and delayed coverage.

Impact on Beneficiaries

Both programs play crucial but distinct roles in the lives of their beneficiaries. Medicaid acts as a safety net for the most vulnerable, often providing more comprehensive coverage for those with limited means. Medicare provides a foundation of healthcare security for older adults and other eligible individuals, helping them navigate health challenges that often come with aging.

Understanding these differences is key to navigating these programs effectively. Whether you're a potential beneficiary, a caregiver, or a healthcare professional, recognizing how Medicaid and Medicare complement and differ from each other is crucial in making informed healthcare decisions.

1.4. Exercise: 10 MCQs with Answers at the End

Let's test your knowledge on Medicaid and Medicare with these multiple-choice questions (MCQs). Try answering them before peeking at the answers at the end!

1. **Medicaid is primarily designed for:**

   A. People over 65

   B. Low-income individuals and families

   C. Veterans

   D. Non-U.S. citizens

2. **Which part of Medicare covers hospital insurance?**

   A. Part A

   B. Part B

   C. Part C

   D. Part D

3. **Medicaid programs are administered by:**

   A. The federal government only

   B. Individual states within federal guidelines

   C. Private insurance companies

   D. The United Nations

4. **Medicare Part D covers:**

   A. Hospital stays

   B. Prescription drugs

   C. Doctor's visits

D. Long-term care

5. **Which of the following is typically covered by Medicaid but not Medicare?**

A. Inpatient hospital services

B. Long-term care

C. Preventive care

D. Hospice care

6. **Medicare eligibility primarily depends on:**

A. Income level

B. Age or certain disabilities

C. Employment history

D. State of residence

7. **Medicaid coverage and eligibility:**

A. Are the same in every state

B. Vary from state to state

C. Are determined by the United Nations

D. Do not exist in the United States

8. Medicare Advantage (Part C) plans:

   A. Are offered by private insurance companies

   B. Replace the need for Part A and Part B

   C. Do not include prescription drug coverage

   D. Both A and B

9. Which of the following individuals would typically be eligible for Medicare?

   A. A 40-year-old with a low income

   B. A 66-year-old retiree

   C. A 30-year-old non-U.S. citizen

   D. A 20-year-old college student

10. Medicaid often has:

   A. High premiums and deductibles

   B. No cost for covered services

   C. Enrollment periods similar to Medicare

   D. The same coverage in all states

Answers:

1. B. Low-income individuals and families

2. A. Part A

3. B. Individual states within federal guidelines

4. B. Prescription drugs

5. B. Long-term care

6. B. Age or certain disabilities

7. B. Vary from state to state

8. D. Both A and B

9. B. A 66-year-old retiree

10. B. No cost for covered services

How did you do? These questions are designed to reinforce your understanding of the key aspects of Medicaid and Medicare, providing a solid foundation as you navigate the rest of this comprehensive guide.

Chapter 2: The History and Evolution of Medicaid and Medicare

2.1. Origins and Development

Let's take a step back in time to explore the origins and development of Medicaid and Medicare, two programs that have profoundly shaped the American healthcare landscape. Like a story unfolding across generations, the history of these programs is a tale of societal needs, political debates, and evolving policies.

The Birth of Medicare

Our story begins in the early 20th century, a time when the concept of health insurance was still in its infancy. The seeds of Medicare were planted during President Franklin D. Roosevelt's era with the Social Security Act of 1935, but it wasn't until 30 years later that these seeds would bear fruit.

Enter President Lyndon B. Johnson and the landmark Social Security Amendments of 1965. Amidst a growing recognition of the healthcare challenges faced by the elderly, these amendments established Medicare, a national health insurance program for Americans aged 65 and older, irrespective of income or medical history. It was a groundbreaking moment, symbolizing a commitment to the health and well-being of the nation's seniors.

Medicaid's Inception

Alongside Medicare, another crucial development took place. Medicaid emerged, crafted to assist those who fell through the cracks of the private insurance market. This program was designed to provide healthcare coverage to low-income individuals and families, complementing Medicare by addressing the needs of a different demographic.

Evolving with Time

From their inception, both Medicare and Medicaid have been dynamic, evolving entities. Their development reflects the changing tides of American social and political thought, economic conditions, and healthcare needs. Over the years, these programs have expanded and adapted, responding to new challenges and shifting demographics.

- In the 1970s and 1980s, amendments were made to improve coverage and accessibility.

- The 1990s saw the introduction of the Medicare Prescription Drug, Improvement, and Modernization Act, paving the way for Part D.

- The early 21st century continued this trend of expansion and refinement, addressing rising healthcare costs and the evolving needs of beneficiaries.

A Continuing Journey

Today, Medicare and Medicaid are not just programs; they are institutions, integral to the fabric of American society. They stand as testaments to the nation's commitment to health and well-being across the lifespan and economic spectrum. As we delve deeper into their histories, remember, these are not just chapters in a book but ongoing stories that touch the lives of millions. The journey of Medicare and Medicaid is far from over, as they continue to adapt and evolve in response to the ever-changing landscape of healthcare and societal needs.

2.2. Major Amendments and Changes

As we continue our historical exploration of Medicaid and Medicare, it's important to highlight the major amendments and changes that have shaped these programs over the years. Like a tree growing and branching out, these programs have expanded and adapted, responding to the needs of an ever-changing society.

Medicare's Milestones

- **1972 Amendments:** A significant leap, this amendment extended Medicare eligibility to individuals under 65 with long-term disabilities and those with End-Stage Renal Disease (ESRD), broadening the program's reach.

- **1980 Omnibus Reconciliation Act:** This introduced the Prospective Payment System (PPS) for hospital payments, a revolutionary step in Medicare's payment methodology, focusing on efficiency and cost-control.

- **Medicare Prescription Drug, Improvement, and Modernization Act of 2003:** Perhaps one of the most substantial changes, this act added Part D, offering prescription drug coverage, a crucial need for many seniors.

- **The Affordable Care Act (ACA) of 2010:** The ACA brought several changes to Medicare, including expanded coverage for preventive care and screenings and a gradual closing of the Part D "donut hole," thereby reducing out-of-pocket costs for prescription drugs.

Transformations in Medicaid

- **Early Expansions:** Initially focused on welfare recipients, Medicaid's eligibility criteria expanded over time to include more low-income Americans, notably pregnant women, children, and individuals with disabilities.

- **Balanced Budget Act of 1997:** This act introduced the State Children's Health Insurance Program (SCHIP), now known as CHIP, extending coverage to children in families with incomes too high for Medicaid but too low for private insurance.

- **The Affordable Care Act (ACA) of 2010:** A landmark change for Medicaid, the ACA proposed expanding Medicaid to all adults with incomes up to 138% of the federal poverty level. While the

Supreme Court made this expansion optional for states, it significantly increased Medicaid's scope in participating states.

- **Recent Developments:** Over the years, various states have taken advantage of waivers to experiment with Medicaid expansion and reforms, tailoring the program to better suit their populations' needs.

An Ongoing Process

These amendments and changes reflect the fluid nature of Medicaid and Medicare, highlighting their ability to adapt in response to societal needs, economic challenges, and healthcare advancements. As we look back at these milestones, it's clear that both programs are not static entities but dynamic and evolving parts of the U.S. healthcare system, continuously shaped by legislative and policy shifts.

In understanding these transformations, we gain a deeper appreciation for how Medicaid and Medicare have become what they are today: robust, multifaceted programs that play a vital role in the health and well-being of millions of Americans.

2.3. Current State and Future Projections

As we turn to the present and gaze into the future, let's examine the current state of Medicaid and Medicare and project what lies ahead. Like peering through a telescope into the horizon, this exploration helps us understand not only where we are but also where we're headed.

The Present Landscape of Medicare

- **Expanded Coverage:** Medicare continues to evolve, offering more comprehensive coverage, including preventive services and telehealth options, increasingly important in today's digital age.

- **Technological Integration:** There's a growing emphasis on integrating technology into Medicare, improving efficiency and patient care through electronic health records and telemedicine.

- **Financial Stability Concerns:** The financial sustainability of Medicare, particularly Part A, is a matter of ongoing concern, with projections indicating potential funding challenges.

Medicare's Road Ahead

- **Aging Population:** As the Baby Boomer generation ages, the number of Medicare beneficiaries is expected to rise significantly, potentially straining the system.

- **Innovative Payment Models:** Efforts to control costs and improve care quality, such as value-based care models, are likely to continue shaping Medicare's structure.

- **Technological and Medical Advancements:** Advances in medicine and technology will necessitate ongoing adaptations in Medicare's coverage and policies.

Current State of Medicaid

- **Expanded Eligibility in Many States:** Following the ACA, many states have expanded Medicaid eligibility, significantly increasing enrollment and providing coverage to a broader segment of the population.

- **Diverse State Approaches:** State-specific innovations and waivers have led to a variety of Medicaid models, addressing unique state demographics and health care needs.

- **Focus on Cost Control and Quality:** States continue to experiment with ways to control costs while improving care quality, including managed care models and community-based care initiatives.

Medicaid's Path Forward

- **Continued Expansion and Reform:** The debate over Medicaid expansion is ongoing, with some states considering expansion and others looking at alternative reforms.

- **Addressing Social Determinants of Health:** There's a growing recognition of the importance of addressing social determinants of health, like housing and nutrition, in Medicaid programs.

- **Sustainability and Flexibility:** Balancing financial sustainability with the need to adapt to changing healthcare landscapes and beneficiary needs will be a key focus.

Concluding Thoughts

The future of Medicaid and Medicare is as dynamic and multifaceted as their past. As these programs continue to adapt to new challenges, demographic shifts, and technological advancements, they remain crucial in the ever-evolving tapestry of American healthcare. Keeping an eye on these developments is essential for beneficiaries, healthcare professionals, and policymakers alike, as they navigate and shape the future of healthcare in the United States.

2.4. Exercise: 10 MCQs with Answers at the End

Test your understanding of the history and evolution of Medicaid and Medicare with these thought-provoking multiple-choice questions. See how well you can navigate the historical waters of these crucial healthcare programs!

1. **Which President signed Medicare and Medicaid into law?**

   A. Franklin D. Roosevelt

   B. John F. Kennedy

   C. Lyndon B. Johnson

   D. Richard Nixon

2. **In what year were Medicare and Medicaid established?**

   A. 1935

   B. 1965

   C. 1980

D. 2003

3. Medicare Part D, which covers prescription drugs, was introduced under which act?

A. Balanced Budget Act of 1997

B. Medicare Prescription Drug, Improvement, and Modernization Act of 2003

C. Affordable Care Act of 2010

D. Social Security Amendments of 1972

4. The State Children's Health Insurance Program (CHIP) was established by the:

A. Omnibus Budget Reconciliation Act of 1989

B. Balanced Budget Act of 1997

C. Medicare Modernization Act of 2003

D. Affordable Care Act of 2010

5. Which of the following is a significant change brought by the Affordable Care Act (ACA) to Medicare?

A. Introduction of Medicare Part C

B. Expansion of Medicaid to all adults in participating states

C. Closing of the Medicare Part D "donut hole"

D. Elimination of Medicare Part B

6. What was the primary focus of the 1980 Omnibus Reconciliation Act for Medicare?

A. Introducing prescription drug coverage

B. Extending eligibility to all low-income individuals

C. Implementing the Prospective Payment System for hospitals

D. Expanding coverage for preventive services

7. Medicaid was initially focused on:

A. All low-income individuals and families

B. Welfare recipients

C. The elderly and disabled

D. Children and pregnant women

8. Medicare Part A is primarily funded through:

A. General tax revenue

B. Premiums paid by beneficiaries

C. The Medicare Trust Fund

D. State governments

9. Which factor is expected to strain Medicare in the future?

A. Decreasing number of beneficiaries

B. Lower healthcare costs

C. Increasing aging population

D. Reduced healthcare technology costs

10. **One key focus for Medicaid's future is:**

A. Eliminating coverage for children

B. Addressing social determinants of health

C. Transitioning to a federal-only program

D. Reducing the number of eligible states

Answers:

1. C. Lyndon B. Johnson

2. B. 1965

3. B. Medicare Prescription Drug, Improvement, and Modernization Act of 2003

4. B. Balanced Budget Act of 1997

5. C. Closing of the Medicare Part D "donut hole"

6. C. Implementing the Prospective Payment System for hospitals

7. B. Welfare recipients

8. C. The Medicare Trust Fund

9. C. Increasing aging population

10. B. Addressing social determinants of health

How did you fare? These questions are designed to reinforce your knowledge of the historical and evolving aspects of Medicaid and Medicare, enriching your understanding of their impact and significance in the American healthcare narrative.

Chapter 3: Eligibility Criteria for Medicaid and Medicare

3.1. Qualifying for Medicaid

Navigating the eligibility criteria for Medicaid can feel like solving a complex puzzle. Each state has its own set of rules within the federal framework, making Medicaid a tapestry of diverse requirements and benefits. Let's unravel this puzzle and understand what it takes to qualify for Medicaid.

Income: The Primary Factor

- **Income Limits:** At its core, Medicaid is for low-income individuals and families. Income limits are set as a percentage of the Federal Poverty Level (FPL) and vary by state and family size.

- **MAGI-Based Method:** Most states use the Modified Adjusted Gross Income (MAGI) method to determine eligibility, which considers taxable income and tax filing relationships.

Categorical Eligibility

- Medicaid isn't just about income; it's also about fitting into specific categories:

  - **Children and Pregnant Women:** They often have higher income eligibility thresholds.

- **Seniors and Individuals with Disabilities:** Eligibility may include considerations beyond income, like medical needs and care requirements.

- **Parents and Caretaker Relatives:** Eligibility often depends on their children's eligibility.

Expanded Medicaid Under the ACA

- **Expansion in Some States:** The Affordable Care Act (ACA) allowed states to expand Medicaid coverage to nearly all adults with incomes up to 138% of the FPL, but not all states have adopted this expansion.

- **Childless Adults:** In states that expanded Medicaid, childless adults can qualify based solely on income, a significant shift from previous rules.

Non-Financial Criteria

- **Residency and Citizenship:** Applicants must be residents of the state where they are applying for Medicaid and either U.S. citizens or certain qualified non-citizens.

- **Other Factors:** Certain assets and resources may be considered, especially for long-term care eligibility.

The Application Process

- **State-Specific:** Each state has its own application process, though most offer online, mail, and in-person options.

- **Documentation:** Applicants typically need to provide proof of income, residency, citizenship, and other relevant information.

Navigating the Complexity

Qualifying for Medicaid can seem daunting due to its varying and intricate criteria. However, understanding these key aspects can significantly ease the process, allowing those in need to access essential healthcare services. Remember, Medicaid is not just a program; it's a pathway to better health and well-being for millions.

3.2. Qualifying for Medicare

While Medicaid qualification can seem like navigating a labyrinth, qualifying for Medicare is more like following a clear, well-marked path. Medicare, primarily based on age or specific medical conditions, has more straightforward eligibility criteria. Let's walk through the key aspects of qualifying for Medicare.

Age-Based Eligibility

- **The Magic Number – 65:** The most common pathway into Medicare is turning 65 years old. It doesn't matter whether you're working, retired, or have sufficient income; age is the primary criterion.

- **Automatic Enrollment:** If you're already receiving Social Security or Railroad Retirement Board benefits before turning 65, you're automatically enrolled in Medicare Parts A and B on the first day of the month you turn 65.

Eligibility for Younger Individuals

- **Disability:** People under 65 can qualify for Medicare if they have been receiving Social Security Disability Insurance (SSDI) for certain disabilities for 24 months.

- **End-Stage Renal Disease (ESRD):** Individuals of any age with ESRD and requiring dialysis or a kidney transplant are eligible.

- **Amyotrophic Lateral Sclerosis (ALS):** Those with ALS (Lou Gehrig's disease) are immediately eligible for Medicare as soon as they begin receiving SSDI benefits.

Medicare Part A: Premium-Free vs. Paid

- **Premium-Free Part A:** Most people don't pay a premium for Part A if they or their spouse paid Medicare taxes while working for at least 10 years (40 quarters).

- **Paid Part A:** If you don't have enough work quarters, you can still buy Part A, but you'll pay a monthly premium.

Medicare Part B: Voluntary Enrollment

- **Part B Enrollment:** Unlike Part A, Part B requires a monthly premium. While it's optional, there is a late enrollment penalty if you don't sign up when you first become eligible but decide to enroll later.

Medicare Part C and D

- **Medicare Advantage (Part C):** For Part C, you must be enrolled in both Parts A and B. Medicare Advantage plans are offered by private insurance companies approved by Medicare.

- **Prescription Drug Coverage (Part D):** Eligibility for Part D requires enrollment in either Part A or B. Part D plans are also offered by Medicare-approved private insurers.

Understanding Enrollment Periods

- **Initial Enrollment Period:** You have a 7-month window around your 65th birthday to sign up for Medicare, which includes the three months before, the month of, and the three months after your birthday.

- **General and Special Enrollment Periods:** If you miss the initial period, there are general and special enrollment periods, but they may involve late penalties.

Qualifying for Medicare is largely a straightforward process based on age, disability status, or specific health conditions. Understanding these eligibility criteria ensures smooth entry into the program, securing your healthcare coverage as you enter your golden years or navigate certain health challenges.

3.3. Special Cases and Exceptions

In the world of Medicaid and Medicare, there are always scenarios that don't quite fit the mold, like puzzle pieces waiting for the right spot. These special cases and exceptions are crucial to understand, as they can significantly impact eligibility and coverage.

Medicaid: Beyond the Standard Criteria

- **Medically Needy Programs:** Some states offer "Medically Needy" programs for those who have significant health needs but exceed the income limits for standard Medicaid. This program allows individuals to "spend down" their excess income on medical bills to qualify.

- **Waivers for Home and Community-Based Services (HCBS):** States may have waivers that provide Medicaid coverage for services to help individuals stay in their homes or community settings, rather than institutional care.

- **Family Planning Services:** Certain states offer Medicaid coverage limited to family planning services for individuals who don't meet traditional eligibility criteria.

- **Breast and Cervical Cancer Program:** Women diagnosed through the CDC's National Breast and Cervical Cancer Early Detection Program may qualify for Medicaid coverage, regardless of income.

Medicare: Navigating Unique Situations

- **Working Past 65:** If you or your spouse are still working and have health insurance through an employer when you turn 65, you can delay enrolling in Medicare Part B without penalty until the employment or coverage ends.

- **Living Abroad:** U.S. citizens living abroad might not qualify for Medicare unless they worked and paid Medicare taxes while abroad or return to live in the U.S.

- **Disability Exceptions:** Certain disabilities, like ALS and ESRD, provide immediate or expedited Medicare eligibility, bypassing the usual 24-month waiting period after receiving SSDI.

Medicare Special Enrollment Periods (SEPs)

- **SEPs for Part C and D:** There are specific circumstances, like moving out of a plan's service area or losing other credible coverage, where you can enroll in or switch Medicare Advantage or Part D plans outside the regular enrollment periods.

- **SEP for Part B:** If you delayed Part B enrollment due to having health coverage through active employment, you have an 8-month SEP to sign up without penalty once employment or the coverage ends.

Understanding Dual Eligibility

- **Medicare and Medicaid:** Some individuals qualify for both Medicare and Medicaid. In these cases, Medicaid can often cover Medicare premiums and out-of-pocket costs, providing comprehensive coverage.

Recognizing these special cases and exceptions is vital in navigating the complex terrain of Medicaid and Medicare. Whether it's finding coverage through a waiver, understanding the impact of working past 65, or managing dual eligibility, these nuances can make a significant difference in accessing and maximizing health care benefits. Being aware of these exceptions ensures that individuals can find the right fit for their unique healthcare needs and circumstances.

3.4. Exercise: 10 MCQs with Answers at the End

Put your knowledge of Medicaid and Medicare eligibility, including special cases and exceptions, to the test with these multiple-choice questions. See how well you've grasped the nuances of these essential healthcare programs!

1. Which group is typically eligible for Medicaid?

A. Individuals over 65 regardless of income

B. High-income families with children

C. Low-income individuals and families

D. Non-U.S. citizens only

2. What is the primary eligibility criterion for Medicare?

A. Being unemployed

B. Reaching the age of 65

C. Having a low income

D. Being a parent

3. **Medicaid's 'Medically Needy' program is designed for:**

   A. Individuals with no medical needs

   B. Those who exceed income limits but have high medical costs

   C. Non-citizens

   D. All seniors over the age of 65

4. **If you are still working at 65 with employer health coverage, you can:**

   A. Never enroll in Medicare

   B. Delay enrolling in Medicare Part B without penalty

   C. Automatically get enrolled in Medicare Part D

   D. Lose all Medicare benefits

5. **Which of the following conditions provides immediate Medicare eligibility?**

   A. High blood pressure

   B. Amyotrophic Lateral Sclerosis (ALS)

   C. Asthma

   D. Arthritis

6. **What does the Medicare Special Enrollment Period allow?**

A. Enrollment in Medicaid

B. Changing Medicare Advantage plans under certain conditions

C. Enrollment in Medicare at any age

D. Waiving all Medicare premiums

7. **Which of the following is a reason for a Special Enrollment Period for Medicare Part D?**

A. Turning 65

B. Losing credible prescription drug coverage

C. Having a high income

D. Living outside the U.S.

8. **Dual eligibility refers to individuals who qualify for:**

A. Both Medicaid and Medicare

B. Medicare Part A and Part B only

C. Medicaid in two different states

D. Both private insurance and Medicaid

9. Home and Community-Based Services (HCBS) waivers under Medicaid are intended to:

A. Provide coverage only for hospitalization

B. Help individuals stay in their homes or community settings

C. Cover international medical expenses

D. Increase premiums for high-income beneficiaries

10. Medicaid coverage for family planning services is:

A. Available in all states

B. Not covered under Medicaid

C. Only for individuals over 65

D. Offered in certain states to those who don't meet traditional criteria

---

Answers:

1. C. Low-income individuals and families

2. B. Reaching the age of 65

3. B. Those who exceed income limits but have high medical costs

4. B. Delay enrolling in Medicare Part B without penalty

5. B. Amyotrophic Lateral Sclerosis (ALS)

6. B. Changing Medicare Advantage plans under certain conditions

7. B. Losing credible prescription drug coverage

8. A. Both Medicaid and Medicare

9. B. Help individuals stay in their homes or community settings

10. D. Offered in certain states to those who don't meet traditional criteria

How did you do? These questions are designed to help reinforce your understanding of the various eligibility criteria and exceptions within Medicaid and Medicare, ensuring a deeper comprehension of these vital healthcare programs.

Chapter 4: Coverage Details: What Medicaid and Medicare Provide

4.1. Understanding Medicaid Coverage

Medicaid, with its diverse and comprehensive coverage, is like a healthcare Swiss Army knife, equipped to handle a wide range of medical needs. However, the specifics of what it covers can vary significantly from state to state. Let's unpack the common elements of Medicaid coverage and explore how they support the health and well-being of beneficiaries.

Mandatory Benefits

- **Hospital Services:** Medicaid covers both inpatient and outpatient hospital services, providing essential care for a range of medical needs.

- **Doctor Visits:** Regular visits to physicians are covered, ensuring beneficiaries have access to necessary medical consultations.

- **Laboratory and X-ray Services:** Essential diagnostic services are included, helping in the accurate diagnosis and management of medical conditions.

- **Nursing Facility Services:** Long-term care in nursing facilities is a crucial component, particularly for elderly and disabled beneficiaries.

- **Home Health Services:** For those who qualify, home health services enable beneficiaries to receive care in their own homes.

Optional Benefits

- **Prescription Drugs:** While most states include prescription drug coverage, the extent and list of covered medications can vary.

- **Physical and Occupational Therapy:** These rehabilitative services are covered by many states, aiding in recovery and improving quality of life.

- **Dental and Vision Services:** Some states offer dental and vision care, though the scope of these services can range widely.

- **Case Management:** This service helps beneficiaries navigate complex health needs and coordinate various types of care.

Special Populations and Services

- **Children's Services:** Medicaid's Early and Periodic Screening, Diagnostic, and Treatment (EPSDT) service ensures children and teenagers receive comprehensive and preventive health care services, including vaccinations, screenings, and dental check-ups.

- **Maternal Health:** Medicaid plays a vital role in covering prenatal and maternity care, supporting the health of both mothers and their babies.

State-Specific Variations

- **Flexibility in Coverage:** States have considerable flexibility in determining which optional benefits to provide, leading to variations in coverage across the country.

- **Benefit Design:** States can also design their benefit packages within federal guidelines, tailoring services to their population's needs.

Impact on Beneficiaries

Medicaid's coverage is broad and impactful, touching the lives of millions. It provides a safety net for the most vulnerable populations, including low-income families, pregnant women, the elderly, and individuals with disabilities. The program plays a critical role in improving access to health care, reducing the financial burden of medical expenses, and enhancing overall public health.

Understanding Medicaid's coverage helps beneficiaries, healthcare providers, and policymakers appreciate the program's scope and limitations. It underscores Medicaid's role as a foundational element of the U.S. healthcare system, continually adapting to meet the evolving needs of its diverse beneficiaries.

4.2. Understanding Medicare Coverage

Medicare, a cornerstone of health care for older Americans and certain younger individuals with disabilities, offers a structured yet comprehensive coverage system. Its various parts are designed to cover a wide range of health care needs, providing a safety net for millions. Let's delve into the details of what Medicare covers.

Medicare Part A: Hospital Insurance

- **Inpatient Hospital Care:** Covers stays in hospitals, including semi-private rooms, meals, general nursing, drugs as part of your inpatient treatment, and other hospital services and supplies.

- **Skilled Nursing Facility Care:** Provides coverage for stays in skilled nursing facilities under certain conditions for a limited time.

- **Hospice Care:** Offers comfort and support for persons with terminal illnesses, including pain relief, symptom management, emotional and spiritual support.

- **Home Health Care:** Covers limited part-time or intermittent skilled nursing care and home health aide services, physical therapy, occupational therapy, and speech-language pathology services.

Medicare Part B: Medical Insurance

- **Doctor's Services:** Covers medically necessary doctor's services, outpatient care, home health services, durable medical equipment, and some preventive services.

- **Preventive Services:** Includes a variety of screenings and tests, like flu shots, diabetes screenings, cancer screenings, and more, aimed at disease prevention and early detection.

- **Outpatient Care:** Covers services you get as an outpatient, including same-day surgery and lab tests.

- **Durable Medical Equipment:** Provides coverage for items like wheelchairs, walkers, and hospital beds for use at home.

Medicare Part C: Medicare Advantage

- **All-in-One Alternative:** These are bundled plans offered by private companies approved by Medicare that typically include Part A, Part B, and usually Part D.

- **Additional Coverage:** May offer extra benefits like vision, hearing, dental, and/or health and wellness programs, which are not covered by Original Medicare.

Medicare Part D: Prescription Drug Coverage

- **Prescription Drugs:** Helps cover the cost of prescription drugs, including many recommended vaccines or shots.

- **Plan Variability:** Coverage and costs vary depending on the plan, with each providing a list of covered drugs (formulary).

Medigap: Supplemental Insurance

- **Gap Coverage:** Medigap policies, sold by private companies, can help pay some of the remaining health care costs that Original Medicare doesn't cover, like copayments, coinsurance, and deductibles.

- **Standardized Plans:** These policies are standardized and are identified in most states by letters.

Understanding Your Coverage

Navigating Medicare's parts can initially seem daunting, but understanding each part's coverage can empower beneficiaries to make informed decisions about their health care. Medicare provides a broad safety net, ensuring that essential health care needs are met, particularly for those in their later years or with specific disabilities. Familiarity with these details is crucial for maximizing the benefits and minimizing out-of-pocket expenses under Medicare.

4.3. Limitations and Exclusions

While Medicaid and Medicare provide extensive coverage, they are not without their limitations and exclusions. Understanding these boundaries is crucial for beneficiaries to effectively navigate their healthcare options and plan for potential out-of-pocket expenses.

Medicaid Limitations and Exclusions

- **Variability by State:** The most significant limitation of Medicaid is the variability in coverage from state to state. What one state may cover extensively, another might limit or exclude.

- **Service Restrictions:** Some states place limits on certain services, such as a cap on the number of covered doctor visits or prescriptions per month.

- **Limited Coverage for Certain Populations:** Certain groups, like childless adults in states that have not expanded Medicaid under the ACA, may find themselves ineligible.

- **Non-Covered Services:** Generally, Medicaid does not cover services like cosmetic surgery, weight loss programs, or adult dental care in many states.

Medicare Limitations and Exclusions

- **Long-Term Care:** Medicare does not cover long-term care (also called Custodial Care), which is a significant limitation for those needing extended nursing home or assisted living care.

- **Routine Dental, Vision, and Hearing:** Original Medicare does not cover routine dental exams, eye exams, eyeglasses, or hearing aids.

- **Overseas Medical Care:** Generally, Medicare does not cover healthcare services you receive outside the United States, with some exceptions.

- **Prescription Drug Coverage:** While Part D covers prescription drugs, there may be limitations based on the plan's formulary, and some medications may not be covered.

Additional Considerations

- **Cost-Sharing and Deductibles:** Both programs involve some level of cost-sharing, like co-payments, coinsurance, and deductibles, which can add up, especially for those with chronic conditions or limited financial resources.

- **Approval for Services:** Certain services may require prior authorization or be subject to medical necessity reviews, which can limit access to some treatments or procedures.

- **Capitation in Managed Care:** In Medicaid and Medicare Advantage plans, the capitation model (fixed amount per enrollee) might influence the availability and approach to certain treatments.

Understanding these limitations and exclusions is vital for beneficiaries to realistically assess what Medicaid and Medicare can offer and what aspects of healthcare they might need to manage through other means, such as supplemental insurance, personal savings, or alternative programs. Being aware of these boundaries ensures that beneficiaries can plan effectively for their healthcare needs and avoid unexpected expenses.

4.4. Exercise: 10 MCQs with Answers at the End

Test your understanding of the coverage, limitations, and exclusions of Medicaid and Medicare with these multiple-choice questions. See how well you grasp the details of these essential health care programs!

1. **Which of the following is a mandatory benefit covered by Medicaid in all states?**

   A. Dental Care for Adults

   B. Inpatient Hospital Services

   C. Weight Loss Programs

   D. Cosmetic Surgery

2. **Medicare Part A does not cover:**

   A. Inpatient hospital care

   B. Skilled nursing facility care

   C. Long-term custodial care

   D. Hospice care

3. **Which is typically not covered by Original Medicare?**

   A. Doctor's visits

   B. Routine eye exams

   C. Inpatient hospital services

   D. Lab tests

4. **Medicaid coverage for prescription drugs:**

   A. Is the same in all states

   B. Varies by state

C. Is not offered by Medicaid

D. Only covers over-the-counter medications

5. **Medicare Part D covers:**

A. Dental care

B. Prescription drugs

C. Overseas medical care

D. Long-term care

6. **Which of the following services is often limited or capped in Medicaid?**

A. Emergency services

B. Number of doctor visits

C. Inpatient hospital services

D. EPSDT services for children

7. **Routine dental care in Medicare is:**

A. Covered under Part A

B. Covered under Part B

C. Covered under Part D

D. Not typically covered

8. Medicare generally does not cover healthcare services:

A. In skilled nursing facilities

B. Received outside the United States

C. In outpatient settings

D. Provided by primary care physicians

9. One limitation of Medicare Part D is:

A. Coverage of all prescription drugs

B. Limitations based on the plan's formulary

C. Unlimited prescription coverage

D. Coverage of medical equipment

10. Medicaid's 'Medically Needy' program allows individuals to qualify by:

A. Spending down their income on medical bills

B. Being over the age of 65

C. Having no medical needs

D. Living in a specific state

Answers:

1. B. Inpatient Hospital Services

2. C. Long-term custodial care

3. B. Routine eye exams

4. B. Varies by state

5. B. Prescription drugs

6. B. Number of doctor visits

7. D. Not typically covered

8. B. Received outside the United States

9. B. Limitations based on the plan's formulary

10. A. Spending down their income on medical bills

How did you do? These questions are designed to help you understand the intricate details of Medicaid and Medicare coverage, including what is and isn't typically covered, aiding you in navigating these vital healthcare programs effectively.

Chapter 5: Enrollment Process for Medicaid and Medicare

5.1. Steps for Medicaid Enrollment

Enrolling in Medicaid might seem daunting, but it's akin to following a recipe – a step-by-step process that leads to a rewarding result. Here's a guide to simplify the Medicaid enrollment process.

Step 1: Determine Eligibility

- **Check State-Specific Criteria:** Since Medicaid is administered by each state, begin by understanding the eligibility criteria in your state.

- **Income and Category Considerations:** Assess whether your income level and category (such as being pregnant, a parent, elderly, or disabled) align with your state's Medicaid requirements.

Step 2: Gather Necessary Documentation

- **Proof of Income:** Collect recent pay stubs, tax returns, or unemployment benefits statements.

- **Identification and Citizenship:** Prepare identification documents like a driver's license, birth certificate, or passport.

- **Additional Documentation:** Depending on your situation, you may need other documents, such as proof of pregnancy, disability, or other health coverage.

Step 3: Complete the Application

- **Choose How to Apply:** Applications can typically be submitted online, by mail, or in person. Online applications are often the quickest method.

- **State-Specific Portals:** Use your state's Medicaid website or the Health Insurance Marketplace at Healthcare.gov for online applications.

- **Fill Out Application Thoroughly:** Ensure all required fields are completed accurately to avoid delays.

Step 4: Submit the Application

- **Online Submission:** If applying online, follow the instructions to submit electronically.

- **Mail or In-Person Submission:** If using mail or in-person methods, ensure all required documents are included and that you keep copies for your records.

Step 5: Await the Determination

- **Processing Time:** The time taken to process Medicaid applications can vary, but states are generally required to provide a decision within 45 days (90 days for disability determinations).

- **Check Status:** Some states allow you to check your application's status online.

Step 6: Review and Understand Your Coverage

- **Notification of Decision:** You'll receive a notification of whether you've been approved or denied.

- **Understand Your Benefits:** If approved, make sure you understand what services are covered and if there are any copayments or restrictions.

Step 7: Regular Renewal

- **Annual Renewal:** Medicaid requires annual renewal to ensure you still qualify. You'll receive a notice about how and when to renew.

Step 8: Update Information as Needed

- **Report Changes:** If there are significant changes in your circumstances (like income, family size, or address), report these to your Medicaid office promptly.

Navigating the Medicaid enrollment process requires attention to detail and an understanding of your state's specific requirements. By following these steps and staying informed about your coverage, you can successfully access the healthcare benefits Medicaid provides.

5.2. Steps for Medicare Enrollment

The journey to enroll in Medicare, while different from Medicaid, is a clearly defined path. By understanding and following the right steps, you can seamlessly navigate the Medicare enrollment process.

Step 1: Determine Your Eligibility

- **Age-Based Eligibility:** Most people become eligible for Medicare when they turn 65. Others may qualify earlier due to disability or specific medical conditions like End-Stage Renal Disease (ESRD) or Amyotrophic Lateral Sclerosis (ALS).

Step 2: Understand Your Enrollment Period

- **Initial Enrollment Period (IEP):** This is a 7-month period that starts three months before the month you turn 65, includes your birth month, and extends three months after.

- **Special Enrollment Period (SEP):** If you're covered under a group health plan based on current employment, you have an SEP to sign up for Part B anytime as long as you or your spouse is working.

Step 3: Decide on Your Medicare Coverage

- **Original Medicare (Part A and B) vs. Medicare Advantage (Part C):** Choose between Original Medicare, which is managed by the federal government, and Medicare Advantage, offered by private insurance companies.

- **Consider Prescription Drug Coverage (Part D):** Decide if you need a separate Part D plan for prescription drugs if you opt for Original Medicare.

Step 4: Prepare to Apply

- **Gather Necessary Documents:** Have your Social Security number and information about your current health insurance and employment handy.

Step 5: Complete the Application

- **Online Application:** The easiest way to apply for Medicare is through the Social Security website.

- **In-Person or Phone Application:** Alternatively, you can apply at your local Social Security office or call Social Security.

Step 6: Await Confirmation

- **Receive Your Medicare Card:** After enrolling, you'll receive your Medicare card in the mail. This usually happens within a few weeks of applying.

- **Review Your Coverage:** Ensure you understand your coverage, including any premiums, deductibles, and co-payments.

Step 7: Consider Additional Coverage

- **Medigap:** If you opt for Original Medicare, you may want to consider a Medigap policy for additional coverage.

- **Review Annually:** Medicare health and drug plans can change annually, so it's a good idea to review your coverage each year during the Open Enrollment Period.

Step 8: Stay Informed

- **Keep Updated:** Be aware of any changes to Medicare, including coverage options and costs, to ensure your health care needs continue to be met.

Enrolling in Medicare is a critical step in ensuring your healthcare needs are covered in your senior years or if you have specific disabilities. By following these steps and staying informed, you can make the most of your Medicare benefits.

5.3. Navigating Enrollment Challenges

Enrolling in Medicaid and Medicare can sometimes feel like navigating through a maze, with various challenges and obstacles along the way. Understanding these potential hurdles and how to overcome them is key to a smooth enrollment process.

Challenges in Medicaid Enrollment

- **Understanding State-Specific Criteria:** Since Medicaid is administered by individual states, the eligibility criteria and coverage can vary widely, potentially leading to confusion.

- **Gathering Required Documentation:** Applicants often face challenges in compiling the necessary documentation, such as proof of income, residency, and citizenship status.

- **Navigating Application Processes:** The complexity of the application process can be daunting, especially for those with limited access to online resources or with language barriers.

- **Delays in Application Processing:** High demand and administrative backlogs can lead to delays in application processing and approval.

Strategies for Medicaid Enrollment Challenges

- **Seek Assistance:** Utilize local community health centers, social workers, or Medicaid offices for help with understanding eligibility and the application process.

- **Organize Documentation:** Keep all required documents organized and readily available to streamline the application process.

- **Follow Up Regularly:** Stay proactive in following up on your application status, especially if you face delays.

Challenges in Medicare Enrollment

- **Understanding Different Parts of Medicare:** The various parts of Medicare (A, B, C, D) and their specific benefits can be complex and confusing to new enrollees.

- **Timing the Enrollment:** Missing the Initial Enrollment Period can lead to penalties and delayed coverage, which can be a significant setback.

- **Choosing Between Original Medicare and Medicare Advantage:** Deciding which type of Medicare to enroll in can be challenging, as each has its pros and cons.

Strategies for Medicare Enrollment Challenges

- **Educate Yourself:** Utilize resources like the official Medicare website, seminars, and counseling services like the State Health Insurance Assistance Program (SHIP) to better understand Medicare.

- **Mark Important Dates:** Keep track of enrollment periods, especially the Initial Enrollment Period, to avoid missing deadlines.

- **Compare Plans:** Thoroughly compare the benefits, costs, and coverage of Original Medicare versus Medicare Advantage plans to determine which best meets your needs.

General Tips for Both Programs

- **Start Early:** Begin the enrollment process as early as possible to allow ample time for research and decision-making.

- **Utilize Online Resources:** Take advantage of online resources and tools provided by both Medicaid and Medicare for easier application and information access.

- **Ask for Help:** Don't hesitate to seek assistance from experts, counselors, or customer service representatives when faced with doubts or challenges.

Navigating the enrollment challenges in Medicaid and Medicare requires patience, organization, and a proactive approach. By understanding these potential hurdles and utilizing available resources and strategies, you can successfully enroll and secure the healthcare coverage you need.

5.4. Exercise: 10 MCQs with Answers at the End

Test your knowledge of the enrollment processes for Medicaid and Medicare with these multiple-choice questions. See if you can navigate through the intricacies of these essential healthcare programs!

1. **What is the first step in enrolling in Medicaid?**

   A. Paying the enrollment fee

   B. Determining eligibility

   C. Selecting a health plan

   D. Applying for Medicare

2. **When does the Initial Enrollment Period for Medicare start?**

   A. At age 60

   B. Three months before turning 65

   C. When you start receiving Social Security benefits

   D. After retiring from work

3. **Medicaid applications can typically be submitted:**

    A. Only in person

    B. Only by mail

    C. Online, by mail, or in person

    D. Through Medicare

4. **Which of the following can lead to delayed processing of Medicaid applications?**

    A. Applying online

    B. High demand and administrative backlogs

    C. Providing all required documentation

    D. Being over the age of 65

5. **What happens if you miss your Initial Enrollment Period for Medicare?**

    A. You can never enroll in Medicare

    B. You may face penalties and delayed coverage

    C. You're automatically enrolled in Medicaid

    D. Your enrollment fees are waived

6. **One key strategy for navigating Medicare enrollment is:**

A. Ignoring the enrollment periods

B. Choosing the first plan you find

C. Educating yourself about the different parts of Medicare

D. Waiting until you need medical care to enroll

7. **For Medicaid, what type of documentation is often required for enrollment?**

A. Travel history

B. Proof of income and residency

C. High school diploma

D. Professional references

8. **What is a Special Enrollment Period in Medicare?**

A. A time to enroll in Medicaid instead

B. A period when premiums are lower

C. A time to enroll without penalty after missing the Initial Enrollment Period under certain conditions

D. A period for changing your name on Medicare records

9. Which strategy can help in navigating Medicaid's enrollment challenges?

A. Delaying the application process

B. Seeking assistance from local community centers or Medicaid offices

C. Avoiding the use of online resources

D. Submitting incomplete documentation

10. What should you do if you experience delays in Medicaid application processing?

A. Withdraw your application

B. Immediately reapply

C. Stay proactive in following up on your application status

D. Assume you are not eligible

Answers:

1. B. Determining eligibility

2. B. Three months before turning 65

3. C. Online, by mail, or in person

4. B. High demand and administrative backlogs

5. B. You may face penalties and delayed coverage

6. C. Educating yourself about the different parts of Medicare

7. B. Proof of income and residency

8. C. A time to enroll without penalty after missing the Initial Enrollment Period under certain conditions

9. B. Seeking assistance from local community centers or Medicaid offices

10. C. Stay proactive in following up on your application status

How well did you do? These questions are designed to help you better understand the enrollment processes and challenges for Medicaid and Medicare, ensuring you're equipped to navigate these essential healthcare programs successfully.

Chapter 6: Medicare Parts Explained: A, B, C, and D

6.1. Medicare Part A: Hospital Insurance

Medicare Part A, often referred to as hospital insurance, is a foundational component of Medicare coverage. It's designed to cover inpatient care in hospitals, skilled nursing facility care, hospice care, and some home health care services. Let's dive into the specifics of what Part A covers and how it works.

Coverage Under Part A

- **Inpatient Hospital Care:** This includes care in a hospital, critical access hospital, or inpatient rehabilitation facility. Coverage typically includes a semi-private room, meals, general nursing, medications as part of your inpatient treatment, and other hospital services and supplies.

- **Skilled Nursing Facility (SNF) Care:** After a qualifying hospital stay, Part A covers certain services in a SNF, like a semi-private room, meals, skilled nursing and rehabilitative services, and other medically necessary services.

- **Hospice Care:** For patients with a terminal illness and a life expectancy of six months or less, Part A covers hospice care, including pain relief, symptom management, and support services.

- **Home Health Care:** Medicare Part A may cover part-time or intermittent skilled nursing care, physical therapy, speech-language pathology services, and continued occupational therapy.

Qualifying for Part A

- Most people age 65 or older are automatically eligible for premium-free Part A if they or their spouse have paid Medicare taxes while working.

- Younger individuals with disabilities, end-stage renal disease (ESRD), or amyotrophic lateral sclerosis (ALS) may also qualify.

Costs Associated with Part A

- **Premium-Free Eligibility:** If you've paid Medicare taxes for a certain length of time (usually 10 years of work), you typically don't pay a monthly premium for Part A.

- **Deductibles and Coinsurance:** While Part A doesn't have a monthly premium for most people, it does have a deductible and coinsurance. The deductible applies to each benefit period, and coinsurance amounts vary based on the length of your hospital or SNF stay.

Understanding Benefit Periods

- A benefit period under Part A begins the day you're admitted as an inpatient in a hospital or skilled nursing facility and ends when you haven't received any inpatient hospital care (or skilled care in a SNF) for 60 days in a row.

Navigating Part A Coverage

- **Enrollment:** If you're receiving Social Security benefits, you're automatically enrolled in Part A. If not, you may need to sign up during your Initial Enrollment Period.

- **Hospital Observation Status:** It's important to know if you're admitted as an inpatient or under observation, as this affects your coverage and out-of-pocket costs.

Medicare Part A plays a crucial role in covering significant health care costs associated with hospitalizations and related care. Understanding the scope of Part A coverage, its costs, and the rules surrounding benefit periods can help beneficiaries effectively manage their health care needs and financial responsibilities.

6.2. Medicare Part B: Medical Insurance

Medicare Part B is often described as medical insurance. It complements Part A by covering two types of services: medically necessary services and preventive services. Let's explore the various aspects of Part B and what it entails for beneficiaries.

Coverage Under Part B

- **Medically Necessary Services:** This includes services or supplies needed to diagnose or treat a medical condition that meet accepted standards of medical practice. It covers things like doctor visits, outpatient care, home health care, durable medical equipment (like wheelchairs), and many preventive services.

- **Preventive Services:** Part B covers many preventive services to prevent illness or detect it at an early stage. This includes services like flu shots, cardiovascular screenings, cancer screenings (such as mammograms and colonoscopies), and diabetes screenings.

Costs Associated with Part B

- **Monthly Premiums:** Most people pay a standard monthly premium for Part B. The premium might be higher based on your income.

- **Annual Deductible and Coinsurance:** Part B also has an annual deductible. After you meet your deductible, you typically pay 20% of the Medicare-approved amount for most doctor services, outpatient therapy, and durable medical equipment.

Enrolling in Part B

- **Automatic Enrollment:** If you're receiving Social Security or Railroad Retirement Board benefits, you'll be automatically enrolled in Part B when you turn 65.

- **Manual Enrollment:** If you're not automatically enrolled, you can sign up during your Initial Enrollment Period, which begins three months before you turn 65 and ends three months after the month you turn 65.

- **Late Enrollment Penalty:** If you don't sign up for Part B when you're first eligible, you may have to pay a late enrollment penalty.

Special Considerations for Part B

- **Employer Coverage:** If you or your spouse is still working and you have health insurance through an employer, you might choose to delay Part B enrollment without penalty.

- **Refusal of Part B:** You can refuse Part B coverage if you don't want it. However, if you decide to enroll later, you may have to pay a late enrollment penalty.

Navigating Part B Coverage

- Understanding the coverage provided by Part B, including preventive services and medically necessary services, is crucial for beneficiaries. It helps in managing healthcare needs and making informed decisions about treatments and medical services.

- Being aware of the costs, such as premiums, deductibles, and coinsurance, and understanding the enrollment process and potential penalties, are essential aspects of managing Part B effectively.

Medicare Part B forms a vital part of the Medicare program, offering coverage for a wide range of medical services and preventive care. Its role in helping beneficiaries manage their healthcare needs is significant, making an understanding of Part B an essential aspect of navigating Medicare.

6.3. Medicare Part C: Medicare Advantage

Medicare Part C, commonly known as Medicare Advantage, offers an alternative way to receive your Medicare benefits. These plans are offered by private insurance companies approved by Medicare and combine Part A, Part B, and often Part D coverage. Let's delve into the details of Medicare Advantage plans and what they entail.

What Medicare Advantage Covers

- **Integrated Coverage:** Medicare Advantage plans include all the benefits of Part A (hospital insurance) and Part B (medical insurance). Most plans also offer prescription drug coverage (Part D).

- **Additional Benefits:** Many plans offer extra benefits that Original Medicare doesn't cover, like dental, vision, hearing, and wellness programs.

- **Annual Out-of-Pocket Limit:** Unlike Original Medicare, Medicare Advantage plans have an annual limit on out-of-pocket expenses for Part A and Part B services.

Types of Medicare Advantage Plans

- **Health Maintenance Organization (HMO) Plans:** Require you to use doctors, hospitals, and other providers within the plan's network.

- **Preferred Provider Organization (PPO) Plans:** Offer more flexibility in choosing providers but often at a higher cost if you go outside the network.

- **Private Fee-for-Service (PFFS) Plans:** Determine how much it will pay providers and how much you must pay when you get care.

- **Special Needs Plans (SNPs):** Tailored for people with specific diseases or characteristics.

Choosing a Medicare Advantage Plan

- **Consider Your Health Care Needs:** Assess your health care needs and preferences, including access to specific doctors or medications.

- **Compare Plans in Your Area:** Look at the costs, coverage, and network of providers for each plan available in your area.

- **Understand Plan Rules:** Be aware of the rules regarding out-of-network services, referrals for specialists, and coverage while traveling.

Enrollment and Costs

- **Eligibility:** To join a Medicare Advantage Plan, you must have Part A and Part B and live in the plan's service area.

- **Enrollment Periods:** You can enroll in a plan during your Initial Enrollment Period when you first become eligible for Medicare, during the Annual Election Period (Oct 15 – Dec 7), or during special enrollment periods if you qualify.

- **Costs:** Costs vary by plan and may include premiums (in addition to your Part B premium), deductibles, and copayments or coinsurance.

Switching Plans and Disenrollment

- **Annual Election Period:** You can switch plans or return to Original Medicare during the Annual Election Period.

- **Medicare Advantage Disenrollment Period:** From January 1 to February 14, you can leave your Medicare Advantage Plan and return to Original Medicare.

Medicare Advantage plans offer a bundled approach to Medicare coverage, often with additional benefits. Understanding the types of plans available, their costs, and the enrollment rules can help beneficiaries make informed decisions that best suit their healthcare needs and preferences.

6.4. Exercise: 10 MCQs with Answers at the End

Test your knowledge of Medicare Parts A, B, C, and D with these multiple-choice questions. This exercise will help reinforce your understanding of the different aspects of Medicare coverage.

1. **Medicare Part A primarily covers:**

   A. Prescription drugs

   B. Outpatient care

   C. Inpatient hospital stays

   D. Dental care

2. **Which of the following is a benefit of Medicare Part B?**

   A. Full coverage for long-term care

   B. Preventive services and doctor's visits

   C. Coverage for overseas medical care

   D. Unlimited prescription drug coverage

3. **Medicare Advantage Plans are also known as:**

   A. Part A

   B. Part B

   C. Part C

   D. Part D

4. **Which type of Medicare Advantage plan generally requires you to use doctors within its network?**

   A. PPO

   B. PFFS

C. HMO

D. SNP

5. What additional benefits might a Medicare Advantage plan offer that Original Medicare does not?

A. Annual out-of-pocket limit

B. Inpatient hospital care

C. Skilled nursing facility care

D. Hospice care

6. To be eligible for Medicare Part C, you must:

A. Be over 65 years old

B. Have both Part A and Part B

C. Have Part D coverage

D. Be eligible for Medicaid

7. Medicare Part D covers:

A. Dental care

B. Prescription drugs

C. Inpatient hospital services

D. Medical equipment

8. Which Medicare part has an annual out-of-pocket limit?

A. Part A

B. Part B

C. Part C

D. Part D

9. What is a key feature of PPO Medicare Advantage Plans?

A. They require referrals for specialists

B. They have a network of preferred providers but still cover out-of-network services

C. They don't cover prescription drugs

D. They are tailored for people with specific diseases

10. During which period can you switch from a Medicare Advantage Plan back to Original Medicare?

A. Initial Enrollment Period

B. Open Enrollment Period for Medicare Advantage

C. Medicare Advantage Disenrollment Period

D. Special Enrollment Period

Answers:

1. C. Inpatient hospital stays

2. B. Preventive services and doctor's visits

3. C. Part C

4. C. HMO

5. A. Annual out-of-pocket limit

6. B. Have both Part A and Part B

7. B. Prescription drugs

8. C. Part C

9. B. They have a network of preferred providers but still cover out-of-network services

10. C. Medicare Advantage Disenrollment Period

How did you do? These questions are designed to help you better understand the different parts of Medicare and the specific coverage options and benefits they provide.

Chapter 7: Medicaid State Variations and Federal Guidelines

7.1. State-Specific Rules and Coverage

One of the unique aspects of Medicaid is the significant variation in how it is administered and the coverage it provides across different states. While adhering to federal guidelines, each state has the flexibility to tailor its Medicaid program to meet the specific needs of its residents. Let's explore these state-specific rules and coverage differences.

Flexibility Within Federal Framework

- **Federal Baseline:** The federal government sets certain baseline requirements and guidelines for all Medicaid programs.

- **State Variations:** States have the discretion to expand their programs beyond these federal minimum standards. This includes broader eligibility criteria, additional services, and different approaches to delivering and managing care.

Eligibility Variations

- **Income Limits:** While all states must follow the basic income eligibility guidelines set by the federal government, they have the latitude to set higher income thresholds, thereby expanding coverage to more residents.

- **Expansion under the ACA:** States have the option to expand Medicaid eligibility to adults under 65 with incomes up to 138% of the federal poverty level. The decision to expand is at the state's discretion, leading to differences in coverage among states.

Covered Services

- **Mandatory vs. Optional Services:** While federal guidelines specify certain mandatory benefits that all Medicaid programs must cover, states can choose to provide additional optional benefits. This results in variations in services like dental care, vision services, prescription drug coverage, and physical therapy.

- **Long-Term Care:** States also differ in how they provide and fund long-term care services, including home and community-based services (HCBS).

Service Delivery Models

- **Managed Care vs. Fee-for-Service:** States can choose to deliver Medicaid services through managed care organizations (MCOs) or a traditional fee-for-service model, or a combination of both. The choice of model can impact how beneficiaries access and receive healthcare services.

Provider Reimbursement Rates

- **Setting Rates:** States set their own provider reimbursement rates within federal guidelines, which can affect the availability of providers participating in Medicaid.

Beneficiary Cost-Sharing

- **Copayments and Premiums:** States have the option to impose copayments, premiums, and other cost-sharing charges on certain Medicaid beneficiaries, within federal limits.

Innovation and Waivers

- **Section 1115 Waivers:** States can apply for waivers to test new or existing ways to deliver and pay for health care services in Medicaid. These waivers allow states to implement programs that may not strictly adhere to federal Medicaid rules.

Understanding the state-specific variations in Medicaid is crucial for beneficiaries, healthcare providers, and policymakers. These variations reflect the diverse needs and priorities of different states and impact how beneficiaries in different regions access and receive healthcare services. It's essential for anyone involved in Medicaid to be aware of the specific rules and coverage details in their respective states to effectively navigate the program.

7.2. The Role of Federal Oversight

While Medicaid programs vary significantly across states, the role of federal oversight remains a critical component in ensuring that these state-run programs adhere to certain national standards and objectives. This federal oversight serves as a balancing act between allowing state flexibility and maintaining consistent, quality healthcare coverage across the country. Let's explore the various facets of this federal oversight in Medicaid.

Setting National Standards

- **Mandatory Benefits and Services:** The federal government mandates certain core benefits that all state Medicaid programs must provide. This ensures a baseline level of healthcare coverage for all Medicaid beneficiaries, regardless of where they live.

- **Eligibility Criteria:** Federal guidelines establish minimum eligibility standards for certain groups, such as low-income families, pregnant women, the elderly, and individuals with disabilities.

Financial Oversight

- **Matching Funds:** The federal government provides a portion of Medicaid funding to states, known as the Federal Medical

Assistance Percentage (FMAP). This matching rate varies by state, based on criteria such as per capita income.

- **Ensuring Proper Use of Funds:** Federal oversight includes monitoring and auditing state Medicaid programs to ensure funds are used appropriately and efficiently.

Quality and Accessibility Standards

- **Ensuring Quality of Care:** The federal government sets standards to ensure a certain level of quality in Medicaid services. These include regulations on provider qualifications, patient rights, and quality assurance measures.

- **Access to Care:** Federal oversight also involves ensuring that Medicaid beneficiaries have sufficient access to healthcare services, which includes monitoring provider networks and service availability.

Promoting Innovation and Flexibility

- **Waivers and Demonstrations:** The Centers for Medicare & Medicaid Services (CMS) grants waivers, such as Section 1115 waivers, allowing states to experiment with different ways of delivering and paying for healthcare. These waivers enable states to tailor their programs to better suit their populations' needs while still adhering to overarching federal goals.

- **Guidance and Support:** The federal government provides guidance, technical assistance, and support to states in implementing and managing their Medicaid programs.

Compliance and Enforcement

- **Ensuring Compliance:** CMS monitors state Medicaid programs for compliance with federal laws and regulations. This includes reviewing state plan amendments and waiver implementations.

- **Enforcement Actions:** When necessary, the federal government can take enforcement actions against states that do not comply with federal Medicaid requirements. These actions can range from financial penalties to other administrative measures.

The role of federal oversight in Medicaid is crucial in maintaining a balance between state autonomy and the need for a cohesive, nationally consistent healthcare safety net. This oversight ensures that despite the variability among state programs, there remains a standard of care and access that all Medicaid beneficiaries can expect.

7.3. Comparing State Medicaid Programs

Comparing Medicaid programs across different states is like looking at a mosaic where each piece has its unique color and texture, yet contributes to a larger picture. The variability in how states design and administer their Medicaid programs can lead to significant differences in coverage, eligibility, and services. Let's explore some key areas where these state Medicaid programs can differ and how these differences impact beneficiaries.

Eligibility Criteria

- **Income Thresholds:** States have flexibility in setting income eligibility levels. Some states have expanded their Medicaid programs under the ACA to cover all adults with incomes up to 138% of the federal poverty level, while others have more restrictive criteria.

- **Asset Tests:** Some states apply asset tests (considering an individual's assets in addition to income) for certain categories of Medicaid applicants, such as the elderly and individuals with disabilities.

Covered Services

- **Mandatory vs. Optional Benefits:** While all states must cover federal mandatory benefits, they have discretion in providing optional benefits. For instance, some states offer more comprehensive dental and vision care, while others may offer limited or no coverage for these services.

- **Long-Term Care:** States vary widely in how they provide and fund long-term care services, particularly in balancing institutional care with home and community-based services.

Service Delivery Models

- **Managed Care vs. Fee-for-Service:** The prevalence of managed care models differs across states. Some states enroll a large portion of their Medicaid population in managed care plans, while others rely more on a fee-for-service model.

- **Innovative Models:** Some states have implemented innovative models like accountable care organizations (ACOs) or patient-centered medical homes to improve care coordination and outcomes.

Provider Participation and Reimbursement Rates

- **Reimbursement Rates:** States set their Medicaid provider reimbursement rates, which can affect the number of providers willing to participate in Medicaid. Higher reimbursement rates generally lead to better provider participation and access for beneficiaries.

- **Provider Networks:** The size and composition of provider networks in Medicaid can vary, impacting beneficiaries' access to specialists and other healthcare services.

Cost-Sharing and Premiums

- **Beneficiary Contributions:** Some states require premiums, deductibles, or copayments for certain Medicaid populations, while others do not. These costs can impact beneficiaries' access to and utilization of healthcare services.

Impact on Beneficiaries

- **Access to Care:** Differences in eligibility, covered services, and provider participation can impact beneficiaries' access to healthcare. For example, beneficiaries in one state may have easier access to specialists or certain types of care compared to those in another state.

- **Quality of Care:** The quality of care in Medicaid can also vary depending on how states manage their programs, including efforts to improve care quality and patient outcomes.

Comparing state Medicaid programs reveals a complex landscape where geography can significantly influence the nature and extent of Medicaid coverage. These variations underscore the importance of understanding your state's specific Medicaid rules and offerings, especially for beneficiaries, policymakers, and healthcare providers who navigate or influence these programs.

7.4. Exercise: 10 MCQs with Answers at the End

Test your understanding of Medicaid's state variations and federal guidelines with these multiple-choice questions. Assess your grasp of how Medicaid programs differ across states and the role of federal oversight.

1. **Medicaid eligibility income thresholds are:**

   A. The same across all states.

   B. Set individually by each state.

   C. Determined by the federal government only.

   D. Based on the national poverty line only.

2. Which of the following is a mandatory benefit that all state Medicaid programs must provide?

A. Dental care for adults

B. Inpatient hospital services

C. Prescription drug coverage

D. Long-term care services

3. The Federal Medical Assistance Percentage (FMAP) is:

A. A fixed percentage for all states.

B. The same as the Medicare reimbursement rate.

C. Different for each state based on criteria like per capita income.

D. Determined by each state's governor.

4. States can use Section 1115 waivers to:

A. Opt out of Medicaid completely.

B. Test new ways of delivering Medicaid services.

C. Increase eligibility thresholds uniformly.

D. Set their own federal matching rate.

5. Medicaid provider reimbursement rates:

A. Are uniform across all states.

B. Vary from state to state.

C. Are set by the federal government.

D. Are the same as Medicare rates.

6. Which optional Medicaid benefit may vary significantly between states?

A. Emergency hospital services

B. Pediatric services

C. Dental care for adults

D. Nursing facility services

7. The primary role of federal oversight in Medicaid is to:

A. Manage day-to-day operations of each state's program.

B. Ensure states comply with national Medicaid standards.

C. Directly pay Medicaid providers.

D. Set specific eligibility criteria for each state.

8. States have the option to expand Medicaid to adults with incomes up to:

A. 100% of the federal poverty level.

B. 138% of the federal poverty level.

C. 200% of the federal poverty level.

D. 250% of the federal poverty level.

9. **State-specific Medicaid programs can differ in:**

A. Federal mandatory benefits they must provide.

B. The balance between institutional care and home and community-based services.

C. The federal matching rate (FMAP).

D. The basic structure of the Medicaid program.

10. **In managing their Medicaid programs, states:**

A. Cannot impose any cost-sharing on beneficiaries.

B. May require premiums, deductibles, or copayments for certain populations.

C. Must provide the same level of benefits as Medicare.

D. Are not allowed to use managed care models.

Answers:

1. B. Set individually by each state.

2. B. Inpatient hospital services

3. C. Different for each state based on criteria like per capita income.

4. B. Test new ways of delivering Medicaid services.

5. B. Vary from state to state.

6. C. Dental care for adults

7. B. Ensure states comply with national Medicaid standards.

8. B. 138% of the federal poverty level.

9. B. The balance between institutional care and home and community-based services.

10. B. May require premiums, deductibles, or copayments for certain populations.

How well did you do? These questions are designed to deepen your understanding of the complexities of Medicaid, including state variations, federal guidelines, and the flexibility states have in administering their programs.

Chapter 8: Medicare Advantage and Supplemental Plans

8.1. Choosing a Medicare Advantage Plan

Selecting a Medicare Advantage (Part C) plan is a significant decision that can affect your healthcare coverage and out-of-pocket costs. Medicare Advantage plans are offered by private insurance companies and provide an alternative to Original Medicare, often including additional benefits. Here's a guide to help you navigate the process of choosing the right Medicare Advantage plan for your needs.

Understand the Types of Medicare Advantage Plans

- **Health Maintenance Organization (HMO):** Typically requires you to use healthcare providers in the plan's network and get referrals for specialists.

- **Preferred Provider Organization (PPO):** Offers more flexibility in choosing providers, with higher costs for out-of-network services.

- **Private Fee-for-Service (PFFS):** The plan determines how much it will pay providers and how much you must pay when you receive care.

- **Special Needs Plans (SNPs):** Tailored to individuals with specific diseases or characteristics, such as chronic illnesses or dual eligibility for Medicaid and Medicare.

Consider Your Healthcare Needs

- **Provider Preferences:** If you have preferred doctors or hospitals, check if they are in the plan's network.

- **Health Conditions:** Consider plans that cater to your specific health needs, especially if you have chronic conditions.

- **Medication Coverage:** Make sure the plan's formulary (list of covered drugs) includes your medications.

Compare Costs and Benefits

- **Premiums, Deductibles, and Copayments:** Evaluate the costs associated with each plan, including out-of-pocket limits.

- **Extra Benefits:** Look for additional benefits that may be important to you, such as dental, vision, hearing, or wellness programs.

- **Quality Ratings:** Medicare provides a star rating system to help compare the quality of Medicare Advantage plans.

Enrollment Periods

- **Initial Enrollment Period:** You can enroll in a Medicare Advantage plan when you first become eligible for Medicare.

- **Annual Election Period (Oct 15 – Dec 7):** You can join, switch, or drop a Medicare Advantage plan during this period each year.

- **Medicare Advantage Open Enrollment Period (Jan 1 – Mar 31):** If you're already enrolled in a Medicare Advantage plan, you can switch to another Medicare Advantage plan or go back to Original Medicare during this period.

Seek Help If Needed

- **Consult Experts:** Utilize resources like State Health Insurance Assistance Programs (SHIP) for free, personalized counseling.

- **Use Medicare's Plan Finder:** Medicare's Plan Finder tool on their website can help you compare plans based on your individual needs.

Choosing a Medicare Advantage plan involves careful consideration of your health needs, financial situation, and the available plan options in your area. By thoroughly evaluating these factors, you can select a plan that best aligns with your healthcare preferences and budget.

8.2. Understanding Supplemental Plans

Medicare Supplemental Insurance, commonly known as Medigap, plays a crucial role in filling the gaps in Original Medicare coverage. These are private insurance policies designed to cover some of the healthcare costs not covered by

Medicare Part A and Part B, such as copayments, coinsurance, and deductibles. Let's explore what Medigap plans cover and how they work.

Basic Features of Medigap Plans

- **Standardized Plans:** There are several standardized Medigap plans available, each labeled with a different letter (e.g., Plan A, Plan B, Plan G). While the benefits in each plan type are standardized across all states (except Massachusetts, Minnesota, and Wisconsin), the costs can vary by insurer.

- **Filling the Gaps:** Medigap plans help pay some of the remaining healthcare costs after Original Medicare (Part A and Part B) pays its share. This can include copayments, coinsurance, and deductibles.

What Medigap Does Not Cover

- **No Additional Services:** Medigap plans generally do not cover long-term care, vision or dental care, hearing aids, eyeglasses, or private-duty nursing.

- **Not a Standalone Policy:** These plans are meant to supplement Original Medicare, not replace it. They don't provide Medicare Part A or Part B benefits.

Choosing a Medigap Plan

- **Assess Your Needs:** Consider your health care needs and financial situation. Look at how often you visit doctors, your regular medications, and your ability to pay out-of-pocket costs.

- **Compare Plans and Costs:** Medigap policies can have different premiums, even for the same benefits. Shop around and compare policies offered by different insurance companies.

- **Enrollment Period:** The best time to buy a Medigap policy is during your 6-month Medigap open enrollment period, which starts the first month you have Medicare Part B and are 65 or older.

State-Specific Differences

- **Variations in Availability:** Not all Medigap plans are available in every state. Additionally, state laws might affect which Medigap policies are available to you if you're under 65 and have Medicare because of disability, end-stage renal disease, or ALS.

Working with Other Insurance

- **Coordination with Other Coverage:** If you have other health insurance, such as employer coverage or Medicaid, it's important to understand how that insurance works with Medicare and Medigap.

- **Cannot Be Used with Medicare Advantage:** You cannot use Medigap insurance to pay for costs in Medicare Advantage Plans (Part C).

Understanding the role of Medigap plans is essential for those enrolled in Original Medicare who need assistance covering out-of-pocket costs. By carefully selecting a Medigap plan that aligns with your healthcare needs and financial capabilities, you can achieve a more comprehensive coverage and reduce financial strain from medical expenses.

8.3. Costs and Benefits Comparison

When considering Medicare options, it's crucial to compare the costs and benefits of different plans, including Original Medicare (Part A and Part B), Medicare Advantage (Part C), and Medigap (Medicare Supplement Insurance) plans. This comparison helps in making an informed decision that aligns with your healthcare needs and financial situation. Let's delve into a comparative analysis of these plans.

Original Medicare (Part A and Part B)

- **Costs:**

  - Part A: Most people don't pay a premium for Part A if they've paid Medicare taxes while working. However, there are deductibles and coinsurance for hospital stays.

  - Part B: Standard monthly premium and an annual deductible, with 20% coinsurance for most services.

- **Benefits:**

  - Covers hospitalization, doctor visits, lab tests, and outpatient procedures.

  - Wide acceptance by doctors and hospitals nationwide.

- **Limitations:**

  - Does not cover prescription drugs, dental, vision, or hearing services.

  - No out-of-pocket maximum.

Medicare Advantage (Part C)

- **Costs:**

  - Varies by plan. Premiums can be low or even $0, but this is in addition to the Part B premium.

  - Usually have copays or coinsurance for services.

- **Benefits:**

  - Often includes prescription drug coverage and may offer additional benefits like dental, vision, and hearing.

  - Out-of-pocket maximum limit.

- **Limitations:**

  - Provider network restrictions (especially for HMO plans).

  - May need referrals for specialists.

Medigap (Medicare Supplement Insurance)

- **Costs:**

  - Additional monthly premium on top of Part B premium.

  - Costs vary by plan and insurer.

- **Benefits:**

  - Helps cover out-of-pocket costs like deductibles and coinsurance.

  - Provides flexibility in choosing providers.

- **Limitations:**

  - Does not include prescription drug coverage – needs to be purchased separately (Part D).

  - No additional benefits like dental or vision.

Costs and Benefits Considerations

- **Budget:** Assess your ability to pay premiums, deductibles, and out-of-pocket costs. Remember that lower premiums might mean higher out-of-pocket costs when you need care.

- **Healthcare Needs:** Consider how often you need medical care, your regular medications, and the need for additional benefits like dental or vision.

- **Provider Preferences:** If you prefer to see certain doctors or specialists, ensure they are covered in the plan's network.

- **Travel:** If you travel frequently, Original Medicare with or without a Medigap plan offers broader coverage across the U.S., while Medicare Advantage plans may have geographic restrictions.

Making a side-by-side comparison of the costs and benefits of each type of Medicare plan can provide a clearer picture of what each option offers and help you make a choice that best suits your healthcare needs and financial capabilities.

8.4. Exercise: 10 MCQs with Answers at the End

Test your understanding of Medicare Advantage and Supplemental Plans with these multiple-choice questions. Evaluate your knowledge of the costs, benefits, and differences between these plans.

1. **Medicare Advantage plans are also known as:**

A. Part A

B. Part B

C. Part C

D. Medigap

2. **Which is typically included in Medicare Advantage (Part C) but not in Original Medicare?**

A. Inpatient hospital services

B. Prescription drug coverage

C. 20% coinsurance on most services

D. Nationwide provider access

3. **Medigap is designed to:**

A. Replace Medicare Part B

B. Cover out-of-pocket costs not covered by Original Medicare

C. Provide prescription drug coverage

D. Serve as a standalone healthcare plan

4. **Which type of plan requires you to use network providers for the lowest costs?**

A. Medigap

B. Original Medicare

C. Medicare Advantage HMO

D. Medicare Part D

5. **An important feature of Medigap policies is that they:**

A. Have an annual out-of-pocket maximum

B. Cover additional services like dental and vision

C. Are standardized across most states

D. Include prescription drug coverage

6. **What is a benefit of Original Medicare (Part A and Part B) over Medicare Advantage plans?**

A. Lower out-of-pocket costs

B. Coverage of prescription drugs

C. Wider acceptance by doctors and hospitals

D. Includes dental and vision coverage

7. Medicare Advantage plans often include:

A. An annual out-of-pocket spending limit

B. Unlimited coverage for all medical services

C. Coverage without any premiums

D. The same benefits nationwide

8. To enroll in a Medigap policy, you must have:

A. Medicare Part C

B. Both Medicare Part A and Part B

C. Only Medicare Part A

D. A prescription drug plan

9. The primary difference between Medicare Advantage PPO and HMO plans is:

A. PPO plans require referrals for specialists

B. HMO plans typically offer more flexibility in choosing providers

C. PPO plans often allow use of out-of-network providers at a higher cost

D. HMO plans have higher premiums

10. **Which statement is true regarding Medicare Advantage plans?**

A. They do not cover any services provided by Original Medicare

B. They are available to individuals without Medicare Part A and Part B

C. They provide an alternative way to receive Medicare benefits, often with additional coverage

D. They always cost more than Original Medicare

Answers:

1. C. Part C

2. B. Prescription drug coverage

3. B. Cover out-of-pocket costs not covered by Original Medicare

4. C. Medicare Advantage HMO

5. C. Are standardized across most states

6. C. Wider acceptance by doctors and hospitals

7. A. An annual out-of-pocket spending limit

8. B. Both Medicare Part A and Part B

9. C. PPO plans often allow use of out-of-network providers at a higher cost

10. C. They provide an alternative way to receive Medicare benefits, often with additional coverage

These questions are aimed at enhancing your understanding of the different aspects of Medicare Advantage and Medigap plans, helping you to make informed decisions about your healthcare coverage.

Chapter 9: Navigating Prescription Drug Coverage

9.1. Medicare Part D Explained

Medicare Part D is a critical component of the Medicare program, providing beneficiaries with prescription drug coverage. This coverage is offered through private insurance plans approved by Medicare. Understanding the intricacies of Part D is essential for effectively managing medication costs and ensuring access to necessary prescriptions.

Overview of Medicare Part D

- **Purpose:** Part D adds prescription drug coverage to Original Medicare, some Medicare Cost Plans, some Medicare Private-Fee-for-Service (PFFS) Plans, and Medicare Medical Savings Account (MSA) Plans.

- **Private Plans:** Part D plans are offered by private insurance companies and can vary in cost and drugs covered.

Choosing a Part D Plan

- **Formulary:** Each Part D plan has its formulary, or list of covered drugs, which is important to review to ensure your medications are covered.

- **Costs:** Costs for Part D plans include premiums, deductibles, copayments, and coinsurance. These costs can vary from plan to plan.

- **Coverage Phases:** Understanding the coverage phases, including the initial deductible, initial coverage, coverage gap (donut hole), and catastrophic coverage, is vital.

Enrollment in Part D

- **Enrollment Periods:** You can enroll in a Medicare Part D plan during your Initial Enrollment Period for Medicare, the Annual Election Period (Oct 15 – Dec 7), or during a Special Enrollment Period if you qualify.

- **Late Enrollment Penalty:** If you don't enroll in Part D when you're first eligible and don't have other creditable prescription drug coverage, you may have to pay a late enrollment penalty.

Coverage Gap ("Donut Hole")

- **Understanding the Donut Hole:** After you and your plan spend a certain amount on covered drugs, you enter the coverage gap, known as the donut hole, where you may pay more for prescription drugs.

- **Out-of-Pocket Threshold:** Once you reach the out-of-pocket spending threshold, you leave the coverage gap and enter the catastrophic coverage phase, where you generally pay significantly less for drugs for the rest of the year.

Factors to Consider

- **Drug Costs:** Consider the cost of drugs under the plan, including whether your medications are on the plan's formulary and at what tier.

- **Pharmacy Network:** Check if your preferred pharmacy is in the plan's network, as this can affect your costs.

- **Plan Ratings:** Medicare provides star ratings for plans based on quality and performance, which can be a helpful tool in selecting a plan.

Medicare Part D plays an indispensable role in making prescription drugs more affordable for Medicare beneficiaries. Navigating its details – from choosing the right plan to understanding the coverage phases – is key to optimizing your prescription drug coverage under Medicare.

9.2. Medicaid Prescription Benefits

Medicaid provides prescription drug coverage as an essential aspect of its comprehensive healthcare benefits, although the specifics can vary from state to state. Understanding how Medicaid handles prescription drug coverage is important for beneficiaries who rely on medications for their health and well-being.

Overview of Medicaid Prescription Drug Coverage

- **Federal Requirements:** While each state has considerable flexibility in designing its own Medicaid prescription drug program, federal law requires states to cover most prescription drugs.

- **State Formularies:** Each state Medicaid program has a formulary, which is a list of covered medications. States decide which drugs to include on their formularies based on effectiveness, safety, and cost-effectiveness.

Coverage and Limitations

- **Mandatory and Optional Drugs:** States are required to cover certain drugs but also have the option to cover additional drugs. Some medications, like cosmetic drugs or weight loss medications, may not be covered.

- **Prior Authorization and Other Restrictions:** States may implement cost-saving measures such as requiring prior authorization, setting quantity limits, or establishing a preferred drug list.

Cost to Beneficiaries

- **Minimal Cost-Sharing:** Medicaid prescription drug coverage typically involves minimal cost-sharing. Some states may charge small copayments, but federal rules limit these charges, especially for certain populations like children and pregnant women.

- **No Cost for Certain Groups:** For some beneficiary groups, like children under the Medicaid Early and Periodic Screening,

Diagnostic, and Treatment (EPSDT) program, prescription drugs are provided at no cost.

Special Considerations

- **Generic vs. Brand-Name Drugs:** Medicaid programs often encourage or require the use of generic drugs when available and medically appropriate, to keep costs down.

- **Managed Care Plans:** Beneficiaries enrolled in Medicaid managed care plans may have different formularies or prescription drug policies compared to those in traditional Medicaid.

Access and Availability

- **Pharmacy Networks:** Beneficiaries typically must obtain medications from pharmacies that are part of the Medicaid program's network.

- **Mail Order and Specialty Pharmacies:** Some states offer or require mail-order services for certain types of medications, like maintenance drugs for chronic conditions.

Understanding the nuances of Medicaid's prescription drug coverage, including what medications are covered, any associated costs, and how to obtain these medications, is crucial for beneficiaries. This knowledge ensures that individuals can effectively access and manage their prescription needs under Medicaid.

9.3. Strategies for Managing Prescription Costs

Managing prescription drug costs is a crucial aspect of healthcare for many individuals, especially those on Medicare or Medicaid. Rising drug prices can pose a significant burden, but there are several strategies that beneficiaries can employ to manage these costs more effectively. Let's explore some practical ways to reduce and manage the cost of prescriptions.

1. Utilize Generic Drugs

- **Opt for Generics:** Whenever possible, choose generic medications. Generics are often much less expensive than brand-name drugs and are equally effective in most cases.

2. Review and Update Medication List with Your Doctor

- **Regular Reviews:** Have regular discussions with your healthcare provider about the medications you're taking. Sometimes, less expensive alternatives or changes in therapy can be equally effective.

- **Medication Effectiveness:** Ensure each medication is still necessary and effective for your condition.

3. Understand Your Prescription Drug Plan

- **Plan Formulary:** Review your Medicare Part D or Medicaid plan's formulary to understand which drugs are covered and at what cost.

- **Tiered Drug Pricing:** Understanding your plan's tiered drug pricing can help you identify lower-cost options.

4. Consider Mail-Order Pharmacies

- **Cost Savings:** Some plans offer lower prices for a larger supply of medication through mail-order pharmacies, which can be particularly beneficial for chronic medications.

5. Use a Preferred Pharmacy Network

- **Lower Copayments:** Some Medicare Part D and Medicaid plans have preferred pharmacy networks that offer medications at lower copayments.

6. Apply for Extra Help or Pharmaceutical Assistance Programs

- **Extra Help Program:** If you have limited income and resources, you may qualify for Medicare's Extra Help program to help pay for prescription drugs.

- **Manufacturer Assistance Programs:** Some pharmaceutical companies offer assistance programs for low-income individuals or those without insurance.

7. Review Annual Changes During Open Enrollment

- **Annual Plan Review:** During the Medicare open enrollment period, review any changes to your plan for the next year and compare with other available plans.

- **Changing Plans:** If another plan offers your medications at a lower cost, consider switching plans.

8. Utilize State Pharmaceutical Assistance Programs (SPAPs)

- **State Programs:** Some states offer pharmaceutical assistance programs that help pay prescription drug costs for eligible residents.

9. Monitor Prescription Drug Usage

- **Track Medications:** Keep track of your medication usage to avoid waste and ensure medications are used efficiently.

10. Consider Therapeutic Alternatives

- **Alternative Therapies:** In consultation with your healthcare provider, explore if there are therapeutic alternatives or over-the-counter options that could be more cost-effective.

By employing these strategies, beneficiaries can better manage their prescription drug costs, ensuring access to necessary medications without undue financial strain. Being proactive and informed about prescription drug coverage and costs is key to effective healthcare management.

9.4. Exercise: 10 MCQs with Answers at the End

Test your understanding of navigating prescription drug coverage with these multiple-choice questions. Assess your grasp of Medicare Part D, Medicaid prescription benefits, and cost management strategies.

1. **Medicare Part D is primarily for:**

   A. Covering long-term care services

   B. Providing hospital insurance

   C. Offering prescription drug coverage

   D. Paying for medical equipment

2. **Which of the following is a common strategy to reduce prescription drug costs?**

   A. Choosing brand-name drugs over generics

   B. Skipping doses to make the prescription last longer

   C. Using mail-order pharmacies for chronic medications

   D. Buying medications from unverified online retailers

3. **Medicaid prescription drug coverage:**

A. Is uniform across all states

B. Varies based on state-specific formularies

C. Does not cover generic drugs

D. Always requires high copayments

4. **The 'donut hole' refers to:**

A. A gap in Medicare Part B coverage

B. The initial deductible phase in Medicare Part D

C. A coverage gap in Medicare Part D where beneficiaries may pay more

D. The catastrophic coverage phase in Medicare Part D

5. **For managing prescription costs, it is advisable to:**

A. Switch to a different medication without consulting a doctor

B. Regularly review and update your medication list with your healthcare provider

C. Use multiple pharmacies to get the best deals

D. Always choose brand-name drugs for better quality

6. **Extra Help is a program that assists with:**

A. Long-term care costs

B. Medicare Part B premiums

C. Prescription drug costs for those with limited income

D. Medical equipment purchases

7. **Preferred pharmacy networks are:**

A. Pharmacies where you can buy non-prescription drugs at a discount

B. Part of Medicare Advantage plans only

C. Pharmacies that offer lower copayments under some Medicare Part D plans

D. Not available under Medicare Part D

8. **State Pharmaceutical Assistance Programs (SPAPs):**

A. Are available in all states

B. Help eligible residents with prescription drug costs

C. Cover all types of medications without restrictions

D. Replace the need for Medicare Part D

9. **A formulary in a prescription drug plan is:**

A. A list of all available medications in the market

B. A list of preferred hospitals and clinics

C. A list of covered drugs under the plan

D. A mandatory federal list of medications for all states

10. **Using generic drugs:**

    A. Is typically discouraged in Medicare Part D plans

    B. Can lead to higher out-of-pocket costs

    C. Is a recommended way to reduce prescription costs

    D. Is not allowed under Medicaid programs

Answers:

1. C. Offering prescription drug coverage

2. C. Using mail-order pharmacies for chronic medications

3. B. Varies based on state-specific formularies

4. C. A coverage gap in Medicare Part D where beneficiaries may pay more

5. B. Regularly review and update your medication list with your healthcare provider

6. C. Prescription drug costs for those with limited income

7. C. Pharmacies that offer lower copayments under some Medicare Part D plans

8. B. Help eligible residents with prescription drug costs

9. C. A list of covered drugs under the plan

10. C. Is a recommended way to reduce prescription costs

These questions are designed to enhance your understanding of the complexities and strategies associated with managing prescription drug coverage under Medicare and Medicaid.

Chapter 10: Dual Eligibility: When You Qualify for Both Medicaid and Medicare

10.1. Understanding Dual Eligibility

Dual eligibility refers to individuals who qualify for both Medicaid and Medicare benefits. This unique status can offer comprehensive health coverage, but it also brings a set of complexities in navigating both programs. Let's delve into what dual eligibility means, who qualifies, and how it works.

Who Are Dual Eligible Beneficiaries?

- **Income and Resource Limits:** Dual eligible individuals typically have low income and limited resources, qualifying them for Medicaid, while also meeting the age or disability requirements for Medicare.

- **Categories:** There are different categories of dual eligibles, including full-benefit dual eligibles who receive the full range of Medicaid benefits, and partial dual eligibles who may receive help with Medicare premiums and cost-sharing.

Types of Dual Eligibility

- **Qualified Medicare Beneficiary (QMB) Program:** Helps pay for Medicare Part A and B premiums, deductibles, coinsurance, and copayments.

- **Specified Low-Income Medicare Beneficiary (SLMB) Program:** Pays for Medicare Part B premiums.

- **Other Programs:** There are additional programs like Qualified Disabled and Working Individuals (QDWI) and Qualified Individuals (QI) that offer specific benefits.

Benefits of Dual Eligibility

- **Comprehensive Coverage:** Dual eligible individuals can receive a wide range of health care services from both Medicare and Medicaid.

- **Cost Savings:** Medicaid can help cover many out-of-pocket costs associated with Medicare, such as premiums, deductibles, and copayments.

- **Extra Services:** Medicaid may cover additional services not provided by Medicare, like long-term care and some dental, vision, and hearing services.

Navigating Dual Eligibility

- **Coordination of Benefits:** It's crucial to understand how Medicare and Medicaid work together. Generally, Medicare serves as the primary payer for covered services, with Medicaid covering remaining eligible costs.

- **Medicare Advantage Plans:** Dual eligibles can choose to enroll in Medicare Advantage plans that are specifically designed for them, known as Special Needs Plans (SNPs).

- **Prescription Drug Coverage:** While Medicare Part D provides prescription drug coverage, Medicaid may cover some drugs and out-of-pocket costs not covered by Medicare.

Enrollment and Assistance

- **Automatic Enrollment:** Some individuals are automatically enrolled in certain Medicaid programs based on their Medicare status.

- **Seeking Help:** State Medicaid offices, SHIP counselors, or social workers can provide assistance and guidance to those navigating dual eligibility.

Understanding dual eligibility is key for beneficiaries who qualify for both Medicaid and Medicare. It offers a pathway to comprehensive healthcare coverage, ensuring that individuals with limited income and resources receive the medical care they need without significant financial burden.

10.2. Coordinating Benefits and Coverage

For individuals who are dual eligible – qualifying for both Medicare and Medicaid – coordinating benefits and coverage between these two programs is crucial. This coordination ensures that healthcare costs are covered in the most efficient and effective manner. Let's explore how benefits and coverage are coordinated for dual-eligible beneficiaries.

Understanding Primary and Secondary Payer

- **Primary Payer:** Medicare typically acts as the primary payer for healthcare services. This means that Medicare pays first for any healthcare services that both Medicare and Medicaid cover.

- **Secondary Payer:** Medicaid usually acts as the secondary payer. After Medicare has paid its share of the costs, Medicaid may cover remaining eligible expenses, such as Medicare deductibles, coinsurance, and copayments.

Coordinating Medical Services

- **Healthcare Providers:** Dual eligible beneficiaries should inform their healthcare providers about their dual status so that billing can be appropriately directed first to Medicare and then to Medicaid.

- **Special Needs Plans (SNPs):** Some Medicare Advantage plans are designed specifically for dual eligibles, offering tailored benefits and provider networks that can facilitate the coordination of services.

Prescription Drug Coverage

- **Medicare Part D:** Dual eligibles are usually enrolled in Medicare Part D for prescription drug coverage. Medicaid may cover certain drugs not included in Medicare Part D plans and can also help with Part D premiums and cost-sharing.

- **Best Available Evidence Policy:** If there is a discrepancy in a dual eligible's Part D plan coverage, the Best Available Evidence policy requires the plan to adjust cost-sharing to the correct amounts based on Medicaid eligibility.

Long-Term Care and Home-Based Services

- **Medicaid's Role:** Medicaid plays a significant role in covering long-term care services, like nursing home care and home and community-based services, which are not typically covered by Medicare.

- **Coordinated Care Models:** Some states have integrated care models to provide more coordinated care for long-term services and supports.

Financial Assistance Programs

- **Medicare Savings Programs (MSPs):** These programs help dual eligibles with Medicare premiums and, in some cases, Medicare deductibles, coinsurance, and copayments.

- **Automatic Enrollment:** Dual eligibles may be automatically enrolled in certain MSPs or the Extra Help program for Medicare Part D.

Avoiding Coverage Gaps

- **Regular Eligibility Reviews:** Dual eligibles should regularly review their eligibility status for both Medicare and Medicaid to avoid any gaps in coverage.

- **Communication with Providers and Plans:** Maintaining open lines of communication with healthcare providers, Medicare, and Medicaid is important for ensuring that all available benefits are utilized effectively.

Coordinating benefits and coverage for dual eligible beneficiaries can be complex, but it's a critical process to ensure comprehensive healthcare coverage and minimize out-of-pocket costs. Understanding how Medicare and Medicaid interact, and utilizing available resources and assistance programs, is key for dual eligibles to effectively manage their healthcare needs.

10.3. Addressing the Challenges of Dual Eligibility

Dual eligibility, where individuals qualify for both Medicaid and Medicare, offers comprehensive health coverage. However, it also comes with unique challenges. Navigating two distinct programs simultaneously can be complex, and beneficiaries often face hurdles in managing their benefits effectively. Let's discuss how to address these challenges.

Understanding Coverage Complexities

- **Navigating Two Systems:** Dual eligibles must understand the specific coverage rules and benefits of both Medicare and Medicaid, which can be daunting due to the varying policies and procedures of each program.

- **Coordination of Benefits:** It's crucial to know which program pays for what and in what order. Medicare typically pays first for covered services, with Medicaid covering remaining costs, but this can vary based on the service.

Accessing Needed Services

- **Provider Networks:** Finding healthcare providers who accept both Medicare and Medicaid can be a challenge, potentially limiting access to care.

- **Service Overlaps and Gaps:** Dual eligibles need to be aware of which services are covered by each program to avoid gaps in coverage, particularly for services like long-term care.

Managing Out-of-Pocket Costs

- **Understanding Cost-sharing:** Dual eligibles often have reduced out-of-pocket costs, but navigating the specifics can be complex, especially with regard to copayments and deductibles.

- **Benefit Maximization:** Ensuring that beneficiaries are taking full advantage of the cost-saving benefits available to them under both programs.

Dealing with Administrative Processes

- **Eligibility and Enrollment:** Keeping up with eligibility criteria, enrollment periods, and renewals for both programs can be challenging.

- **Paperwork and Documentation:** Managing the paperwork and documentation requirements for each program can be overwhelming for some beneficiaries.

Strategies for Addressing Challenges

- **Seek Assistance:** Beneficiaries can seek help from resources like State Health Insurance Assistance Programs (SHIP), Medicaid offices, or social workers.

- **Stay Informed:** Keeping up-to-date with changes in both Medicare and Medicaid policies is crucial.

- **Regularly Review Coverage:** Periodically reviewing coverage and benefits under both programs helps in understanding and utilizing the benefits effectively.

- **Leverage Community Resources:** Community organizations and advocacy groups can provide support and guidance in managing dual eligibility.

Integrated Care Programs

- **Special Needs Plans (SNPs):** Some Medicare Advantage plans are designed specifically for dual eligibles and can help streamline care coordination.

- **PACE Programs:** Programs of All-Inclusive Care for the Elderly (PACE) are another option in some areas, offering comprehensive medical and social services.

Addressing the challenges of dual eligibility involves a combination of staying informed, seeking appropriate assistance, and carefully managing healthcare services and benefits. For many beneficiaries, overcoming these challenges is key to accessing the full range of benefits available to them, ensuring comprehensive and cost-effective healthcare coverage.

10.4. Exercise: 10 MCQs with Answers at the End

Test your knowledge about dual eligibility for Medicaid and Medicare with these multiple-choice questions. This exercise will help you understand the intricacies of navigating both programs as a dual eligible beneficiary.

1. **Dual eligibility refers to individuals who are eligible for:**

   A. Medicare only

   B. Medicaid only

   C. Both Medicare and Medicaid

   D. Neither Medicare nor Medicaid

2. **What does Medicare typically cover as the primary payer for dual eligibles?**

   A. Long-term care

   B. Prescription drugs

   C. All healthcare services

   D. Copayments and deductibles

3. **Medicaid acts as a _ payer, covering costs not paid by Medicare for dual eligibles.**

    A. Primary

    B. Secondary

    C. Sole

    D. Tertiary

4. **Which program typically helps dual eligibles with Medicare Part B premiums?**

    A. Qualified Medicare Beneficiary (QMB) Program

    B. Special Needs Plans (SNPs)

    C. Medicaid Expansion under the ACA

    D. Medicare Part D Extra Help

5. **One of the challenges for dual eligibles is:**

    A. Finding providers who accept both Medicare and Medicaid

    B. Automatic disqualification from Medicaid

    C. Increased out-of-pocket costs

    D. Mandatory enrollment in Medicare Advantage

6. **Which of these is a resource for dual eligibles to navigate their benefits?**

A. Private insurance brokers

B. State Health Insurance Assistance Programs (SHIP)

C. Federal Trade Commission

D. National Institutes of Health

7. **For dual eligibles, Medicare often covers _ and Medicaid may cover _ .**

A. Prescription drugs; long-term care

B. Long-term care; prescription drugs

C. All healthcare services; none

D. None; all healthcare services

8. **Special Needs Plans (SNPs) in Medicare Advantage are specifically designed for:**

A. All senior citizens

B. Individuals with specific diseases

C. Dual eligibles

D. High-income beneficiaries

9. The Qualified Medicare Beneficiary (QMB) program helps dual eligibles with:

A. Medicaid premiums

B. Medicare Part A and B premiums

C. Food and housing assistance

D. Employment opportunities

10. Which factor complicates healthcare access for dual eligibles?

A. High premiums for Medicaid

B. Simplified enrollment processes

C. Limited provider networks accepting both Medicare and Medicaid

D. Mandatory participation in clinical trials

Answers:

1. C. Both Medicare and Medicaid

2. C. All healthcare services

3. B. Secondary

4. A. Qualified Medicare Beneficiary (QMB) Program

5. A. Finding providers who accept both Medicare and Medicaid

6. B. State Health Insurance Assistance Programs (SHIP)

7. A. Prescription drugs; long-term care

8. C. Dual eligibles

9. B. Medicare Part A and B premiums

10. C. Limited provider networks accepting both Medicare and Medicaid

These questions are intended to enhance your understanding of the complexities faced by individuals who are dual eligible for Medicaid and Medicare, and the resources available to help navigate these challenges.

Chapter 11: Financial Aspects: Understanding Costs and Payments

11.1. Medicaid Costs and Contributions

Medicaid is designed to provide health care coverage to low-income individuals and families, but understanding the costs and contributions associated with Medicaid is important for beneficiaries. Let's explore the financial aspects of Medicaid, including any costs that beneficiaries may be responsible for.

Medicaid Costs for Beneficiaries

- **Minimal or No Premiums:** In most cases, Medicaid beneficiaries do not have to pay premiums. Some states may charge premiums, particularly for certain groups like higher-income beneficiaries or those in Medicaid expansion populations.

- **Copayments:** While Medicaid costs are generally much lower than private insurance, some beneficiaries may have to pay copayments for certain services. These copayments are typically modest and are capped by federal regulations to ensure affordability.

- **No Cost for Certain Groups:** Certain populations, such as children, pregnant women, and individuals receiving long-term care, are often exempt from copayments.

State Variations in Cost-Sharing

- **Varied Policies:** States have flexibility in setting cost-sharing policies within federal guidelines, leading to variations in copayment amounts and the services for which they are charged.

- **Income-Based Scaling:** In some states, cost-sharing requirements for Medicaid beneficiaries are scaled based on income, with higher-income beneficiaries potentially paying higher copayments.

Contributions for Long-Term Care

- **Asset Assessment:** For long-term care coverage under Medicaid, an individual's assets may be assessed. In some cases, individuals may need to spend down their assets to qualify.

- **Estate Recovery:** Federal law requires states to seek reimbursement from the estates of certain Medicaid beneficiaries for long-term care costs paid by Medicaid.

Medicaid Spend-Down Programs

- **Medically Needy Pathway:** Some states have "medically needy" or "spend-down" programs for individuals who have significant health expenses but whose income is too high to qualify for Medicaid under other eligibility groups.

- **Reducing Countable Income:** These programs allow individuals to "spend down" their excess income on medical bills to meet the Medicaid income eligibility requirement.

Understanding and Managing Medicaid Costs

- **Stay Informed:** Beneficiaries should understand their state's specific Medicaid policies regarding premiums, copayments, and spend-down programs.

- **Seek Assistance:** If there are concerns about affording care or understanding cost-sharing requirements, beneficiaries should seek assistance from Medicaid offices, social workers, or community health advocates.

Medicaid's goal is to minimize the financial burden of healthcare for low-income individuals and families. While there may be some costs involved for beneficiaries, these are generally designed to be affordable and manageable, ensuring that essential healthcare services remain accessible to those who need them most.

11.2. Medicare Premiums and Deductibles

Understanding the financial aspects of Medicare, specifically the premiums and deductibles associated with its various parts, is crucial for beneficiaries. These costs can significantly impact a beneficiary's budget, so it's important to be aware of them. Let's break down the premiums and deductibles for Medicare Parts A, B, and D.

Medicare Part A Costs

- **Premiums:** Most beneficiaries don't pay a monthly premium for Part A (hospital insurance) if they or their spouse paid Medicare taxes while working for a certain period (usually 10 years).

- **Deductible:** Part A has a deductible for each benefit period, which covers hospital stays and other inpatient services.

- **Coinsurance:** There are also coinsurance costs for extended hospital and skilled nursing facility stays.

Medicare Part B Costs

- **Premiums:** Part B (medical insurance) comes with a monthly premium. The standard premium amount can change annually and may be higher based on income.

- **Deductible:** There is an annual deductible for Part B, after which you typically pay 20% of the Medicare-approved amount for most doctor services, outpatient therapy, and durable medical equipment.

- **Income-Related Monthly Adjustment Amount (IRMAA):** Higher-income beneficiaries may pay an IRMAA, an extra amount in addition to the standard Part B premium.

Medicare Part D Costs

- **Premiums:** Part D (prescription drug coverage) premiums vary by plan. Like Part B, there may be an IRMAA for beneficiaries with higher incomes.

- **Deductible:** Plans may have a deductible, which varies.

- **Copayments or Coinsurance:** After meeting the deductible, beneficiaries pay copayments or coinsurance for their medications until they reach the out-of-pocket threshold that leads to catastrophic coverage.

Additional Considerations

- **Annual Changes:** Medicare costs can change each year, so it's important to review any updates during the open enrollment period.

- **Late Enrollment Penalties:** If you don't sign up for Part B or Part D when you're first eligible, you may have to pay a late enrollment penalty, which can increase your premiums.

Understanding these costs associated with Medicare Parts A, B, and D is essential for budgeting and financial planning. Beneficiaries should regularly review their Medicare costs and coverage options, particularly during annual enrollment periods, to ensure they are making the most cost-effective choices for their healthcare needs.

11.3. Navigating Payment Systems

For beneficiaries of Medicaid and Medicare, understanding and navigating the payment systems of these programs can be complex. These systems determine how healthcare providers are reimbursed for services, which can impact the availability and delivery of care. Let's delve into the payment systems for Medicaid and Medicare, and how beneficiaries can effectively navigate them.

Medicare Payment Systems

- **Fee-for-Service (Original Medicare):** Under Parts A and B, Medicare typically pays providers a set fee for each service or procedure. Beneficiaries are responsible for deductibles and coinsurance.

- **Medicare Advantage (Part C):** These plans, offered by private insurers, receive a fixed payment per enrollee from Medicare and may have different cost-sharing structures.

- **Part D Payment:** For prescription drugs under Part D, payment varies by plan, with beneficiaries typically paying a portion of drug costs through deductibles, copayments, or coinsurance.

Medicaid Payment Systems

- **State-Defined Rates:** Medicaid payment rates for services are set by each state within federal guidelines. Rates can vary widely between states.

- **Managed Care:** Many states use managed care systems, where Medicaid pays a fixed amount per enrollee to a managed care organization (MCO), which then pays providers.

- **Fee-for-Service (FFS):** In states that use FFS models, Medicaid pays providers directly for each service, similar to Medicare's FFS system.

Navigating the Payment Systems as a Beneficiary

- **Understand Your Coverage:** Know what services are covered under your plan and the associated cost-sharing responsibilities.

- **Provider Networks:** For Medicare Advantage and Medicaid MCOs, it's important to use providers within the plan's network to minimize costs.

- **Billing and Reimbursement:** Be aware of how billing works for your plan. In FFS models, providers bill Medicare or Medicaid directly. In managed care, billing is typically handled by the MCO.

- **Medigap for Medicare:** If you have Original Medicare, consider a Medigap policy to help cover out-of-pocket costs that Medicare doesn't pay.

- **Seek Assistance:** If you have questions about billing or payment, contact your Medicare plan, Medicaid office, or a counselor from a State Health Insurance Assistance Program (SHIP).

Understanding the Impact on Care

- **Provider Participation:** Payment rates can influence which providers participate in Medicare and Medicaid, affecting beneficiaries' access to care.

- **Service Availability:** Payment systems can also impact the types of services available, particularly under managed care plans.

Navigating the payment systems of Medicaid and Medicare requires a clear understanding of how these systems work and how they impact your healthcare coverage. By staying informed and proactive, beneficiaries can ensure they are maximizing their benefits while minimizing out-of-pocket costs.

11.4. Exercise: 10 MCQs with Answers at the End

Test your understanding of the financial aspects of Medicaid and Medicare, including costs, contributions, and payment systems, with these multiple-choice questions. This exercise will help you navigate the complexities of managing healthcare expenses under these programs.

1. **Most beneficiaries do not pay a premium for Medicare Part A because:**

   A. They are over 65 years old

   B. They or their spouse paid Medicare taxes while working

   C. They have a low income

   D. Part A does not cover important services

2. **Medicare Part B premiums are:**

   A. The same for all beneficiaries

   B. Based on income level

   C. Always free

   D. Determined by state governments

3. **For Medicaid, copayments:**

   A. Are the same across all states

   B. Vary depending on the state's policies

   C. Are always higher than Medicare copayments

   D. Do not exist in Medicaid

4. **Which of the following is a feature of Medicare Advantage (Part C) payment system?**

A. Fee-for-service

B. Fixed payment per enrollee

C. Payment based on income

D. Standardized rates across all states

5. **Medicaid's 'spend-down' program is for individuals who:**

A. Have no income

B. Have high medical expenses relative to their income

C. Are dual eligible

D. Want to enroll in Medicare

6. **Medicare Part D prescription drug plans:**

A. Have uniform costs across all plans

B. Include costs like premiums, deductibles, and copayments

C. Are free for all beneficiaries

D. Cover all prescription drugs without restrictions

7. **The Medicare Part A deductible is applied:**

A. Once per year

B. For each hospital stay

C. Monthly

D. For each doctor's visit

8. In Medicaid, states set provider reimbursement rates that:

A. Are the same for all providers

B. Vary between states

C. Are determined by the federal government

D. Match Medicare rates

9. Which program helps low-income individuals with Medicare Part D costs?

A. Medicaid

B. Extra Help

C. Medigap

D. State Pharmaceutical Assistance Programs (SPAPs)

10. Medicare Part B's coinsurance typically requires beneficiaries to pay:

A. A fixed amount per service

B. 20% of the Medicare-approved amount for most services

C. All costs out-of-pocket

D. The full amount until the deductible is met

Answers:

1. B. They or their spouse paid Medicare taxes while working

2. B. Based on income level

3. B. Vary depending on the state's policies

4. B. Fixed payment per enrollee

5. B. Have high medical expenses relative to their income

6. B. Include costs like premiums, deductibles, and copayments

7. B. For each hospital stay

8. B. Vary between states

9. B. Extra Help

10. B. 20% of the Medicare-approved amount for most services

These questions are designed to help you better understand the financial aspects of Medicaid and Medicare, including how costs are determined and managed, and how these affect beneficiaries.

Chapter 12: Legal and Ethical Considerations in Health Care

12.1. Rights and Responsibilities of Beneficiaries

Beneficiaries of healthcare programs like Medicaid and Medicare have specific rights and responsibilities. These rights are designed to protect beneficiaries, while responsibilities ensure the effective and ethical use of healthcare services. Understanding these rights and responsibilities is crucial for beneficiaries to navigate the healthcare system effectively.

Rights of Beneficiaries

- **Right to Information:** Beneficiaries have the right to receive clear and accurate information about their coverage, including what is covered, how to get services, and what costs they must pay.

- **Right to Privacy:** Beneficiaries' personal and health information must be kept private, and they have the right to know who has access to their records.

- **Right to Fair Treatment:** All beneficiaries are entitled to fair and equal treatment without discrimination based on race, color, national origin, disability, age, or gender.

- **Right to Appeal:** Beneficiaries have the right to appeal any decision about their coverage or services. This includes the right to ask for a review of decisions that deny, reduce, or stop services.

- **Right to Quality Care:** Beneficiaries are entitled to receive quality healthcare that is necessary and appropriate for their condition.

Responsibilities of Beneficiaries

- **Providing Accurate Information:** Beneficiaries are responsible for providing accurate and complete information to the best of their knowledge to healthcare providers and program administrators.

- **Understanding Their Coverage:** Beneficiaries should understand their health coverage, including knowing their benefits, limitations, and the costs they are responsible for.

- **Following Prescribed Treatments:** Beneficiaries are expected to follow the treatments and instructions provided by their healthcare providers.

- **Reporting Fraud and Abuse:** Beneficiaries have a responsibility to report any suspected fraud or abuse in the healthcare system.

- **Respecting Health Care Providers:** Beneficiaries should respect healthcare providers and their policies, including appointment times and office protocols.

Navigating Rights and Responsibilities

- **Education and Advocacy:** Beneficiaries can seek information and assistance from program administrators, patient advocates, or legal representatives to better understand and exercise their rights.

- **Active Participation:** Being actively involved in one's healthcare, including participating in treatment decisions and understanding the implications of those decisions, is an essential part of being a responsible beneficiary.

Understanding and exercising these rights and responsibilities helps ensure that beneficiaries receive the healthcare they need while contributing to the integrity and sustainability of healthcare programs. This knowledge empowers beneficiaries to be more effective advocates for their own health and well-being.

12.2. Legal Framework Governing Medicaid and Medicare

Medicaid and Medicare, as major healthcare programs in the United States, operate within a comprehensive legal framework. This framework establishes the rules, regulations, and guidelines under which these programs operate, ensuring they serve their intended purpose while protecting the rights of beneficiaries. Let's explore the key legal aspects governing Medicaid and Medicare.

Foundational Laws and Amendments

- **Social Security Act:** Both Medicaid and Medicare were established under the Social Security Act. Medicare was introduced as part of the Act in 1965, providing health insurance to people aged 65 and older. Medicaid, introduced in the same year, was designed to provide healthcare coverage to low-income individuals and families.

- **Subsequent Amendments:** Over the years, numerous amendments have been made to expand, modify, and improve these programs, adapting them to changing healthcare needs and societal dynamics.

Regulatory Authorities

- **Centers for Medicare & Medicaid Services (CMS):** CMS, a federal agency within the Department of Health and Human Services (HHS), administers Medicare, Medicaid, and other health programs. CMS develops rules and regulations, provides oversight, and ensures compliance with the statutory requirements.

- **State Administration of Medicaid:** While Medicaid is a federal program, it is administered by individual states within federal guidelines. States have some flexibility in determining eligibility, benefits, and payment structures.

Compliance and Enforcement

- **Regulatory Compliance:** Healthcare providers, insurers, and beneficiaries must comply with a myriad of rules and regulations to participate in Medicaid and Medicare.

- **Fraud and Abuse Prevention:** Laws such as the False Claims Act and Anti-Kickback Statute are crucial in combating fraud and abuse in these programs. CMS and other federal and state agencies actively work to identify and prevent fraudulent activities.

Beneficiary Protections

- **Appeals and Grievances:** The legal framework provides beneficiaries the right to appeal decisions and file grievances regarding their coverage, treatment, or care.

- **Privacy and Security:** Laws like the Health Insurance Portability and Accountability Act (HIPAA) protect the privacy and security of beneficiaries' health information.

Quality and Accessibility Standards

- **Quality Assurance:** Legal requirements ensure that Medicaid and Medicare services meet certain quality standards. These include provider qualifications, health and safety standards, and the efficacy of treatments.

- **Accessibility and Non-Discrimination:** Laws like the Americans with Disabilities Act (ADA) and provisions in the Affordable Care Act (ACA) ensure that Medicaid and Medicare services are accessible to all eligible individuals without discrimination.

Understanding the legal framework of Medicaid and Medicare is essential for beneficiaries, healthcare providers, and policymakers. This framework not only governs how the programs operate but also establishes the rights and protections of those they serve, ensuring that these vital healthcare services are delivered fairly, efficiently, and effectively.

12.3. Ethical Issues in Health Care Coverage

Health care coverage, particularly in programs like Medicaid and Medicare, often intersects with various ethical issues. These ethical considerations can range from questions of equitable access to treatment decisions and resource allocation. Understanding these ethical dimensions is crucial for policymakers, healthcare providers, and beneficiaries. Let's explore some of the key ethical issues in health care coverage.

Equitable Access to Care

- **Equality vs. Equity:** There's an ongoing debate about how to ensure that all individuals have equal access to healthcare services, considering factors like income, geography, and social determinants of health.

- **Coverage for Underserved Populations:** Ensuring that vulnerable and underserved populations receive adequate healthcare coverage remains a significant ethical challenge.

Allocation of Limited Resources

- **Cost vs. Care:** Balancing the cost of healthcare with the need to provide comprehensive and quality care is a persistent ethical dilemma. This includes decisions about which treatments and drugs are covered and to what extent.

- **Prioritization of Services:** Determining how to prioritize limited resources, such as in the case of organ transplants or new and expensive treatments, involves complex ethical considerations.

Patient Autonomy and Decision Making

- **Informed Consent:** Ensuring that patients have the necessary information to make informed decisions about their care, and respecting their choices, is a fundamental ethical principle.

- **End-of-Life Care:** Decisions around end-of-life care, including the extent of treatment and palliative care options, involve sensitive ethical considerations, particularly regarding patient autonomy and quality of life.

Privacy and Confidentiality

- **Data Protection:** Safeguarding patient information and ensuring confidentiality in the era of electronic health records is a key ethical concern.

- **Balancing Privacy and Care Coordination:** Finding the right balance between protecting patient privacy and sharing information for better care coordination and treatment is a nuanced ethical issue.

Impact of Social Determinants of Health

- **Addressing Inequalities:** Understanding and addressing how social determinants like housing, education, and employment impact health care access and outcomes is an ongoing ethical challenge.

- **Program Design and Implementation:** Ethically designing and implementing health care programs to effectively address these social determinants is critical.

Responsibility and Accountability

- **Provider Ethics:** Healthcare providers face ethical considerations in delivering care within the constraints of coverage programs, balancing patient needs with program rules and limitations.

- **Systemic Accountability:** There's a broader ethical responsibility for the healthcare system, including government and private insurers, to operate transparently, equitably, and effectively.

Navigating these ethical issues requires a careful balance of legal, moral, and social considerations. For individuals involved in healthcare decision-making, whether at the policy, provider, or personal level, awareness of these ethical dimensions is crucial in making informed, conscientious decisions.

12.4. Exercise: 10 MCQs with Answers at the End

Test your understanding of the legal and ethical considerations in health care, particularly as they relate to Medicaid and

Medicare. These questions will help assess your grasp of the rights, responsibilities, legal frameworks, and ethical issues associated with these health care programs.

1. The primary legislation that established Medicare and Medicaid is the:

A. Affordable Care Act

B. Health Insurance Portability and Accountability Act (HIPAA)

C. Social Security Act

D. Medicare Modernization Act

2. Which agency oversees the administration of Medicare and Medicaid?

A. The Department of Health and Human Services (HHS)

B. The Centers for Medicare & Medicaid Services (CMS)

C. The Federal Trade Commission (FTC)

D. The Centers for Disease Control and Prevention (CDC)

3. One of the key ethical issues in healthcare coverage is:

A. Profit maximization

B. Equitable access to care

C. Advertising strategies

D. Technology development

4. **An ethical dilemma in healthcare resource allocation is:**

A. Deciding who should receive high-cost treatments

B. Choosing the location of new hospitals

C. Determining executive salaries

D. Selecting healthcare advertisement themes

5. **In the context of Medicare and Medicaid, patient autonomy is primarily concerned with:**

A. Patients' ability to pay for services

B. Patients' right to make informed decisions about their care

C. The speed at which patients receive care

D. The choice of healthcare providers by patients

6. **The False Claims Act is significant in healthcare because it:**

A. Regulates drug prices

B. Addresses fraud and abuse in healthcare programs

C. Sets standards for electronic health records

D. Defines healthcare quality metrics

7. **Medicaid beneficiaries' right to privacy is protected under:**

A. The Affordable Care Act

B. The Medicare Modernization Act

C. The Health Insurance Portability and Accountability Act (HIPAA)

D. The Social Security Act

8. An important responsibility of healthcare beneficiaries is to:

A. Report suspected fraud and abuse

B. Participate in healthcare policymaking

C. Ensure profitability of healthcare providers

D. Manage healthcare facilities

9. Social determinants of health primarily refer to:

A. Genetic factors influencing health

B. Lifestyle choices impacting health

C. Economic and social conditions affecting health

D. Hospital locations and their accessibility

10. In healthcare, the concept of 'informed consent' is essential for:

A. Ensuring financial transparency

B. Allowing patients to make decisions based on understanding risks and benefits

C. Healthcare provider training

D. Legal compliance with insurance policies

Answers:

1. C. Social Security Act

2. B. The Centers for Medicare & Medicaid Services (CMS)

3. B. Equitable access to care

4. A. Deciding who should receive high-cost treatments

5. B. Patients' right to make informed decisions about their care

6. B. Addresses fraud and abuse in healthcare programs

7. C. The Health Insurance Portability and Accountability Act (HIPAA)

8. A. Report suspected fraud and abuse

9. C. Economic and social conditions affecting health

10. B. Allowing patients to make decisions based on understanding risks and benefits

These questions are designed to enhance your understanding of the legal and ethical considerations in Medicaid and Medicare, highlighting the complexities and responsibilities involved in navigating these health care programs.

Chapter 13: Technology in Medicaid and Medicare

13.1. The Impact of Digital Transformation

The integration of technology in Medicaid and Medicare is reshaping how these programs operate and interact with beneficiaries, providers, and the healthcare system at large. This digital transformation is improving efficiency, accessibility, and the quality of healthcare services. Let's explore the various impacts of this digital shift.

Enhanced Access to Information

- **Online Portals and Apps:** Beneficiaries can access their healthcare information, manage appointments, and communicate with providers through digital platforms like MyMedicare.gov and state Medicaid websites.

- **Easier Benefit Management:** Technology simplifies the management of benefits, including checking coverage details, tracking claims, and reviewing treatment histories.

Improved Data Management and Analytics

- **Electronic Health Records (EHRs):** The widespread adoption of EHRs has facilitated better coordination of care, reduced duplicative tests, and improved treatment outcomes.

- **Data Analytics:** Advanced analytics are being used to monitor program performance, improve service delivery, and detect fraud and abuse.

Telehealth and Remote Monitoring

- **Expanded Telehealth Services:** Both Medicaid and Medicare have expanded coverage for telehealth services, providing beneficiaries with remote access to healthcare, especially critical in rural or underserved areas.

- **Remote Patient Monitoring:** Technologies that allow for remote monitoring of patients' health can lead to better chronic disease management and preventive care.

Streamlining Administrative Processes

- **Automation and AI:** Automation and artificial intelligence are being used to streamline administrative tasks, reduce paperwork, and enhance decision-making processes.

- **Electronic Billing and Claims Processing:** These technologies improve the efficiency and accuracy of billing and claims processing, reducing administrative burdens for providers and payers.

Enhancing Fraud Detection and Compliance

- **Advanced Fraud Detection Tools:** Technology enables more effective detection of fraudulent activities and non-compliance through sophisticated data analysis.

- **Compliance Monitoring:** Digital tools assist in ensuring that providers and beneficiaries comply with program rules and regulations.

Challenges and Considerations

- **Cybersecurity:** With the increase in digital data, ensuring the security and privacy of health information is a major concern.

- **Digital Divide:** There is a need to address the digital divide, ensuring that all beneficiaries, regardless of their technological capabilities or access, can benefit from these advancements.

The digital transformation in Medicaid and Medicare is revolutionizing the landscape of these programs. By leveraging technology, these programs are enhancing the efficiency and quality of healthcare delivery, although it's crucial to balance these advancements with considerations of security, privacy, and equitable access.

13.2. E-Health and Telemedicine in Medicare and Medicaid

E-health and telemedicine have become increasingly important components of healthcare delivery in Medicare and Medicaid programs. These technologies enable remote healthcare services, providing convenience, accessibility, and often, cost savings. Let's delve into how e-health and telemedicine are integrated into these programs and their impact on healthcare delivery.

Telemedicine in Medicare and Medicaid

- **Expanding Access:** Telemedicine significantly expands access to healthcare, especially for beneficiaries in rural areas, those with mobility issues, or in situations like the COVID-19 pandemic.

- **Services Offered:** Telehealth services in these programs can include virtual consultations, remote patient monitoring, and telepsychiatry, among others.

Medicare and Telehealth

- **Coverage Expansion:** Medicare has increasingly broadened its coverage for telehealth services, especially in response to the COVID-19 pandemic. This includes a wider range of services and allowing beneficiaries to receive telehealth services from their homes.

- **Provider Availability:** Medicare beneficiaries can access telehealth services from various providers, including doctors, nurse practitioners, clinical psychologists, and licensed clinical social workers.

Medicaid and Telehealth

- **State-Specific Policies:** Medicaid telehealth policies are determined at the state level, leading to variability in the extent and types of covered telehealth services.

- **Innovative Programs:** Some Medicaid programs have implemented innovative telehealth programs, such as remote monitoring for chronic diseases and telemedicine kiosks in underserved areas.

Benefits of E-Health and Telemedicine

- **Convenience and Safety:** Telehealth offers convenient access to healthcare services from home, reducing travel time and exposure to pathogens in clinical settings.

- **Continuity of Care:** It facilitates continuity of care, allowing patients to maintain regular contact with their healthcare providers.

- **Cost-Effectiveness:** Telehealth can be cost-effective, reducing the need for certain in-person services and potentially lowering healthcare costs.

Challenges and Barriers

- **Technology Access:** Access to necessary technology and reliable internet remains a barrier for some beneficiaries, particularly in rural or low-income areas.

- **Reimbursement Policies:** Navigating reimbursement policies for telehealth services can be complex, with variations in coverage between Medicare and Medicaid.

- **Privacy and Security:** Ensuring the privacy and security of health information during telehealth sessions is crucial.

Looking Ahead

- **Policy Evolution:** As the benefits of telehealth become more evident, both Medicare and Medicaid are likely to continue evolving their policies to incorporate more e-health services.

- **Integration into Healthcare:** Ongoing integration of telemedicine into standard healthcare practices is anticipated, making remote healthcare a regular component of patient care.

E-health and telemedicine in Medicare and Medicaid represent significant strides in modernizing healthcare delivery, improving access, and potentially enhancing patient outcomes. As technology continues to evolve, these programs are likely to further embrace digital healthcare solutions.

13.3. Future Trends in Health Care Technology

The landscape of healthcare technology is rapidly evolving, and these advancements are poised to significantly influence the future of health care, including in Medicaid and Medicare. Let's explore some key trends that are expected to shape healthcare technology in the coming years.

1. Artificial Intelligence (AI) and Machine Learning

- **Predictive Analytics:** AI will increasingly be used for predictive analytics in healthcare, helping to anticipate patient needs, identify risk factors, and prevent diseases.

- **Diagnostic Tools:** AI-driven diagnostic tools are expected to become more prevalent, offering more accurate and quicker diagnoses.

2. Personalized Medicine

- **Genomics and Precision Treatments:** Advances in genomics will lead to more personalized medicine, where treatments and medications are tailored to individual genetic profiles.

- **Wearable Technology:** The use of wearable devices to monitor health indicators will support personalized healthcare plans and preventive medicine.

3. Expansion of Telehealth Services

- **Broader Adoption:** The use of telehealth services is expected to expand beyond virtual visits to include a wider range of remote healthcare services.

- **Integration with Traditional Care:** Telehealth will become more seamlessly integrated with traditional in-person healthcare delivery.

4. Blockchain in Healthcare

- **Secure Data Sharing:** Blockchain technology could revolutionize how health data is shared and secured, enhancing interoperability and privacy.

- **Fraud Prevention:** Blockchain has the potential to significantly reduce fraud and abuse in healthcare systems, including Medicaid and Medicare.

5. Internet of Medical Things (IoMT)

- **Connected Devices:** The proliferation of connected medical devices will enhance patient monitoring and data collection, improving treatment outcomes and patient care.

- **Remote Patient Monitoring:** IoMT will play a critical role in remote patient monitoring, particularly for chronic disease management.

6. Enhanced Cybersecurity Measures

- **Data Protection:** As healthcare becomes more digitized, robust cybersecurity measures will be crucial to protect sensitive health information.

- **Compliance with Regulations:** Ensuring compliance with healthcare regulations like HIPAA will be essential in the adoption of new technologies.

7. 3D Printing in Medicine

- **Customized Medical Equipment:** 3D printing technology will be used to create customized medical devices and implants tailored to individual patients.

- **Pharmaceutical Applications:** There is potential for 3D printing to be used in creating personalized dosages of medications.

8. Augmented and Virtual Reality

- **Medical Training:** AR and VR will be increasingly used for medical training and education, providing immersive and interactive learning experiences.

- **Patient Rehabilitation:** These technologies will also find applications in patient rehabilitation and therapy.

The future of healthcare technology is promising, with potential to improve patient outcomes, enhance efficiency, and reduce costs. As these technologies develop, Medicaid and Medicare will need to adapt and evolve to incorporate these innovations effectively into their programs.

13.4. Exercise: 10 MCQs with Answers at the End

Test your knowledge of the emerging trends in healthcare technology and their impact on Medicaid and Medicare. These questions will help you understand the current and future role of technology in enhancing healthcare delivery.

1. **Artificial Intelligence in healthcare is primarily used for:**

   A. Replacing human doctors

   B. Predictive analytics and diagnostics

   C. Physical therapy

   D. Performing surgeries

2. **Personalized medicine in healthcare involves:**

   A. Standard treatment for all patients

   B. Treatments tailored to individual genetic profiles

   C. Focus on group therapies

   D. One-size-fits-all medication dosages

3. **The expansion of telehealth services is expected to include:**

A. Only virtual doctor visits

B. A wider range of remote healthcare services

C. Reduced use of technology in healthcare

D. Elimination of in-person visits

4. **Blockchain technology in healthcare can be used for:**

A. Speeding up surgical procedures

B. Secure data sharing and fraud prevention

C. Direct patient care

D. Replacing electronic health records

5. **The Internet of Medical Things (IoMT) refers to:**

A. An internet service exclusively for doctors

B. Connected medical devices enhancing patient monitoring

C. Online medical gaming platforms

D. Virtual reality applications in surgery

6. **A key benefit of enhanced cybersecurity measures in healthcare is:**

A. Faster internet speeds

B. Protection of sensitive health information

C. Increased use of paper records

D. Reduced need for patient consent

7. **3D printing in medicine is NOT currently used for:**

A. Creating customized medical devices

B. Pharmaceutical applications

C. Replacing human organs

D. Making personalized implants

8. **Augmented and Virtual Reality in healthcare are used for:**

A. Only entertaining patients

B. Medical training and patient rehabilitation

C. Billing and coding

D. Performing remote surgeries

9. **A major challenge in the adoption of new healthcare technologies is:**

A. Ensuring entertainment value

B. Balancing technology with traditional practices

C. Avoiding any digital use

D. Limiting patient interaction

10. **In the future, wearable technology in healthcare will primarily be used for:**

   A. Fashion purposes

   B. Personalized health monitoring and preventive medicine

   C. Replacing doctors

   D. Monitoring weather patterns

Answers:

1. B. Predictive analytics and diagnostics

2. B. Treatments tailored to individual genetic profiles

3. B. A wider range of remote healthcare services

4. B. Secure data sharing and fraud prevention

5. B. Connected medical devices enhancing patient monitoring

6. B. Protection of sensitive health information

7. C. Replacing human organs

8. B. Medical training and patient rehabilitation

9. B. Balancing technology with traditional practices

10. B. Personalized health monitoring and preventive medicine

These questions are designed to help you better understand the evolving role of technology in healthcare, particularly in relation to Medicaid and Medicare, and the potential impacts of these technological advancements.

Chapter 14: Planning for the Future: Long-Term Care and End-of-Life Decisions

14.1. Medicaid and Medicare in Long-Term Care

Long-term care involves a variety of services designed to meet a person's health or personal care needs during a short or long period. Understanding how Medicaid and Medicare cover long-term care is crucial for effective planning. Let's explore their roles in providing long-term care services.

Medicare's Coverage of Long-Term Care

- **Limited Coverage:** Medicare primarily covers short-term care for rehabilitation or recovery, such as skilled nursing facility care following a hospital stay. It does not cover long-term custodial care (care that helps with activities of daily living).

- **Home Health Services:** Medicare can cover home health services like intermittent skilled nursing care, physical therapy, and occupational therapy, under certain conditions.

Medicaid's Coverage of Long-Term Care

- **Broader Coverage:** Medicaid is the primary source of payment for long-term care services in the United States, including both institutional care (like nursing homes) and home and community-based services (HCBS).

- **Eligibility Requirements:** Eligibility for Medicaid long-term care services requires meeting certain income and asset limits, which vary by state.

Community and Home-Based Services (HCBS)

- **Medicaid Waivers:** Many states use Medicaid waivers to provide HCBS for individuals who would otherwise be eligible for institutional care. These services can include personal care, home health aides, and respite care.

- **Focus on Independence:** HCBS are designed to help individuals stay in their homes and communities, promoting independence and quality of life.

Considerations in Long-Term Care Planning

- **Assessment of Needs:** Understanding the level of care required, whether it's skilled care or custodial care, is crucial in determining the appropriate long-term care services.

- **Financial Planning:** Given the high costs associated with long-term care, financial planning is essential. This may involve considering private long-term care insurance, personal savings, or exploring eligibility for Medicaid.

- **Legal Considerations:** Planning for long-term care might involve legal considerations like setting up advance directives or exploring options like trusts for asset management.

End-of-Life Care

- **Medicare Hospice Benefits:** For end-of-life care, Medicare offers hospice benefits, which cover comprehensive comfort care for patients with a terminal illness and a life expectancy of six months or less.

- **Medicaid Benefits:** Medicaid also covers hospice care, and in some states, it may provide additional end-of-life services through HCBS waivers.

Planning for long-term care is a critical aspect of healthcare management, especially for older adults and individuals with chronic conditions or disabilities. Understanding how Medicaid and Medicare can support these needs is essential for making informed decisions about care and preparing for the future.

14.2. Making Informed End-of-Life Decisions

End-of-life decisions are some of the most personal and significant choices individuals can make about their healthcare. These decisions often involve considering various medical, ethical, and personal factors. Understanding the options and implications of end-of-life care is crucial for making informed choices that align with an individual's values and wishes. Let's discuss key aspects of making informed end-of-life decisions.

Understanding End-of-Life Care Options

- **Hospice Care:** Focuses on comfort and quality of life, rather than curative treatment, for individuals with a terminal illness and a life expectancy of six months or less.

- **Palliative Care:** Provides relief from the symptoms and stress of a serious illness, with a goal to improve quality of life for both the patient and the family.

Advance Directives and Planning

- **Living Wills:** A legal document that outlines an individual's preferences regarding medical treatments in the event they become unable to communicate their decisions.

- **Health Care Power of Attorney (POA):** Appoints a person to make healthcare decisions on behalf of the individual if they are unable.

Considerations in Decision-Making

- **Personal Values and Beliefs:** Decisions should reflect the individual's values, beliefs, and preferences regarding end-of-life care.

- **Medical Factors:** Understanding the medical aspects of one's condition and the potential outcomes of different treatments is essential.

- **Communication with Healthcare Providers:** Open discussions with healthcare providers about prognosis, treatment options, and what to expect can aid in decision-making.

The Role of Family and Loved Ones

- **Involvement in Planning:** Including family members in discussions about end-of-life care can ensure that everyone understands the individual's wishes.

- **Support and Advocacy:** Family members can provide support and advocate on behalf of the individual to ensure their wishes are respected.

Legal and Ethical Considerations

- **Respecting Patient Autonomy:** It's important to respect the individual's right to make their own decisions about end-of-life care.

- **Navigating Ethical Dilemmas:** Healthcare providers and families often face ethical dilemmas, especially when the patient's wishes are unknown or unclear.

Utilizing Resources and Support

- **Counseling and Support Services:** Many healthcare providers offer counseling and support services to help individuals and families navigate end-of-life decisions.

- **Educational Resources:** Utilizing resources to understand the nature of various end-of-life care options can be helpful.

Making informed end-of-life decisions involves careful consideration of a wide range of factors. It is a deeply personal process that requires thoughtful planning, clear communication, and respect for the individual's values and wishes. Ensuring that these decisions are well-informed and documented can provide peace of mind and clarity during challenging times.

14.3. Preparing for Future Health Care Needs

Preparing for future healthcare needs is an essential aspect of long-term health planning, particularly as it pertains to aging and potential changes in health status. Effective preparation involves considering a range of factors from financial planning to understanding available healthcare services. Let's explore the key steps in preparing for future healthcare needs.

Assessing Potential Health Care Needs

- **Anticipate Changes:** Consider potential health changes that might occur with aging or as a result of chronic conditions.

- **Understand Family Health History:** Knowing your family health history can help anticipate future healthcare needs.

Financial Planning for Health Care

- **Estimate Costs:** Consider the costs of potential healthcare needs, including long-term care, and plan accordingly.

- **Explore Insurance Options:** Understand what is covered by Medicare, Medicaid, or private insurance, and consider purchasing long-term care insurance if needed.

Legal and Medical Planning

- **Advance Directives:** Prepare legal documents like living wills and healthcare proxies to ensure your healthcare wishes are respected.

- **Regular Medical Check-ups:** Regular check-ups and preventive care can help in early detection and management of health issues.

Lifestyle Considerations

- **Healthy Living:** Adopting a healthy lifestyle, including a balanced diet, regular exercise, and avoiding harmful habits, can reduce the risk of chronic diseases.

- **Social Connections:** Maintaining social connections and mental stimulation is vital for mental and emotional health.

Understanding Medicare and Medicaid Benefits

- **Know Your Benefits:** Familiarize yourself with Medicare and Medicaid benefits, including what services are covered and how to access them.

- **Stay Informed on Changes:** Keep abreast of any changes in Medicare and Medicaid policies that might affect your coverage.

Long-Term Care Planning

- **Explore Long-Term Care Options:** Understand the different types of long-term care services available, including home care, assisted living, and nursing home care.

- **Consider Location and Accessibility:** Think about where you want to receive care and whether your current home is suitable for aging in place.

Seek Professional Advice

- **Consult Health Care Professionals:** Regularly discuss your health status and future needs with healthcare providers.

- **Financial and Legal Advisors:** Seek advice from financial planners and legal advisors to ensure comprehensive planning.

Preparing for future healthcare needs is a multifaceted process that requires thoughtful consideration of health, lifestyle, financial, and legal aspects. By taking proactive steps and staying informed, you can ensure that your healthcare needs will be well-managed in the future, allowing for peace of mind and better quality of life.

14.4. Exercise: 10 MCQs with Answers at the End

Test your knowledge on long-term care, end-of-life decisions, and preparing for future health care needs with these multiple-choice questions. This exercise is designed to help you understand the complexities and considerations involved in these important aspects of health care planning.

1. **Long-term care in Medicaid primarily covers:**

   A. Short-term hospital stays

   B. Prescription drugs only

   C. Nursing home care and home-based services

   D. Cosmetic surgeries

2. **A living will is a legal document that:**

   A. Details a person's financial will

   B. Outlines end-of-life care preferences

   C. Assigns legal guardianship

   D. Manages retirement funds

3. **Medicare typically covers long-term custodial care:**

   A. Fully and without restrictions

   B. Only in nursing homes

   C. Not at all

   D. At a 50% cost-share

4. **One aspect of preparing for future healthcare needs is:**

   A. Avoiding regular medical check-ups

   B. Understanding family health history

   C. Ignoring lifestyle changes

   D. Purchasing only short-term health insurance

5. **Financial planning for healthcare primarily involves:**

   A. Estimating future travel expenses

   B. Planning for potential healthcare costs

   C. Investing in stocks and bonds

   D. Buying luxury items

6. **Advance directives are important because they:**

   A. Direct how to invest for healthcare

   B. Ensure financial stability

   C. Ensure an individual's healthcare wishes are known

   D. Are legally required for all adults

7. **The primary role of Medicare in end-of-life care is providing:**

   A. Hospice benefits

   B. Long-term rehabilitation

   C. Permanent residence in nursing homes

D. Unlimited prescription drugs

8. **Healthy lifestyle choices in preparing for future healthcare needs include:**

   A. Regular exercise and balanced diet

   B. Decreasing social interactions

   C. Increasing sedentary activities

   D. Focusing solely on physical health

9. **A healthcare proxy is a person who:**

   A. Manages healthcare investments

   B. Makes medical decisions on behalf of someone if they are unable

   C. Provides home care services

   D. Works exclusively in hospitals

10. **In long-term care planning, it's important to consider:**

   A. Only immediate health needs

   B. Location and accessibility of care

   C. Avoiding all insurance products

   D. Disregarding legal advice

Answers:

1. C. Nursing home care and home-based services

2. B. Outlines end-of-life care preferences

3. C. Not at all

4. B. Understanding family health history

5. B. Planning for potential healthcare costs

6. C. Ensure an individual's healthcare wishes are known

7. A. Hospice benefits

8. A. Regular exercise and balanced diet

9. B. Makes medical decisions on behalf of someone if they are unable

10. B. Location and accessibility of care

These questions are intended to deepen your understanding of the various aspects involved in planning for long-term care, making end-of-life decisions, and preparing for future healthcare needs.

Chapter 15: Navigating Changes and Challenges in Medicaid and Medicare

15.1. Keeping Up with Policy Changes

Medicaid and Medicare are dynamic programs that undergo regular policy changes. These changes can impact coverage, costs, and eligibility, making it essential for beneficiaries, healthcare providers, and policymakers to stay informed. Let's explore effective ways to keep up with these policy changes.

Staying Informed on Policy Updates

- **Official Websites and Newsletters:** Regularly visit official websites like Medicare.gov and CMS.gov, and subscribe to their newsletters for the latest updates.

- **State Medicaid Websites:** For Medicaid, check your state's Medicaid website, as state-specific changes can significantly impact coverage and services.

Utilizing Government Resources

- **State Health Insurance Assistance Programs (SHIP):** These programs provide free, local, one-on-one insurance counseling and assistance to Medicare beneficiaries.

- **Social Security Administration:** They provide information on how changes in Medicare and Medicaid can affect Social Security benefits.

Engaging with Health Care Providers

- **Regular Consultations:** Discuss any changes in Medicaid and Medicare policies during appointments to understand how they might affect your care.

- **Provider Bulletins and Communications:** Many healthcare providers also share updates with patients, especially about changes that may impact services and billing.

Participating in Community and Advocacy Groups

- **Community Organizations:** Local community organizations often host informational sessions on changes in healthcare policies.

- **Advocacy Groups:** Organizations that advocate for seniors or people with disabilities can be valuable resources for information and guidance.

Monitoring Legislative Developments

- **Follow News Outlets:** Stay updated on healthcare legislation and policy discussions through reputable news sources.

- **Legislative Alerts:** Subscribe to legislative alerts from advocacy organizations related to healthcare.

Impact of Policy Changes

- **Coverage and Benefits:** Be aware of how changes might affect your current healthcare coverage and benefits.

- **Eligibility Requirements:** Changes in policy could alter eligibility requirements for both Medicaid and Medicare.

- **Cost Implications:** New policies can impact premiums, deductibles, and out-of-pocket expenses.

Preparing for Changes

- **Review Annual Notices:** Pay attention to the Annual Notice of Change (ANOC) letter if you are enrolled in a Medicare Advantage or Part D plan.

- **Financial Planning:** Adjust your healthcare budgeting based on anticipated or confirmed policy changes.

Keeping up with policy changes in Medicaid and Medicare requires proactive engagement and utilization of available resources. By staying informed, beneficiaries can make the best decisions for their healthcare needs and ensure they maximize their benefits under these programs.

15.2. Addressing Common Challenges

Beneficiaries of Medicaid and Medicare often encounter a range of challenges, from navigating complex program rules to dealing with coverage gaps. Understanding these challenges and knowing how to address them is crucial for effective healthcare management. Let's discuss some common challenges and strategies to overcome them.

Complexity of Program Rules

- **Challenge:** Both Medicaid and Medicare have intricate rules and regulations that can be difficult to understand.

- **Solution:** Utilize resources like SHIP counselors, Medicaid offices, or online tools provided by CMS to help understand program specifics.

Coverage Gaps

- **Challenge:** There can be gaps in what Medicaid and Medicare cover, particularly for services like long-term care, dental, vision, and hearing aids.

- **Solution:** Consider supplemental insurance policies, like Medigap for Medicare beneficiaries, or explore other insurance options to fill these gaps.

Changing Health Needs

- **Challenge:** As beneficiaries age or their health status changes, their healthcare needs can evolve, necessitating different coverage.

- **Solution:** Regularly assess healthcare needs and adjust Medicare or Medicaid plans accordingly. Explore options like Medicare Advantage plans or Medicaid waivers that might better suit changing needs.

Eligibility Issues

- **Challenge:** Changes in income or personal circumstances can affect eligibility for Medicaid and certain parts of Medicare.

- **Solution:** Stay informed about eligibility requirements and report any changes in circumstances promptly to ensure continuous coverage.

Cost Concerns

- **Challenge:** Beneficiaries often face concerns about the costs of premiums, deductibles, and copayments.

- **Solution:** Explore assistance programs like Medicare Savings Programs or Medicaid's spend-down programs to help manage costs.

Access to Providers

- **Challenge:** Finding healthcare providers that accept Medicaid or Medicare, especially in certain specialties or locations, can be challenging.

- **Solution:** Use Medicare and Medicaid's online provider directories to find participating healthcare providers. Consider telehealth options where available.

Medication Coverage

- **Challenge:** Coverage for certain medications can be limited, and costs can be high.

- **Solution:** Review the formulary of Medicare Part D plans or Medicaid to ensure necessary medications are covered. Explore pharmaceutical assistance programs for additional support.

Administrative Burdens

- **Challenge:** Dealing with paperwork, appeals, and billing can be overwhelming.

- **Solution:** Seek assistance from healthcare advocates, social workers, or legal aid services for help with administrative tasks.

Staying Informed

- **Challenge:** Keeping up with changes in Medicaid and Medicare policies and regulations.

- **Solution:** Regularly check official websites, subscribe to newsletters, and attend informational workshops or webinars.

Addressing these common challenges in Medicaid and Medicare requires a combination of staying informed, seeking appropriate assistance, and being proactive in healthcare management. By understanding and tackling these challenges, beneficiaries can ensure they receive the healthcare services they need while minimizing financial strain.

15.3. Advocacy and Seeking Assistance

Navigating Medicaid and Medicare can often be complex, and beneficiaries may sometimes need assistance or advocacy to fully benefit from these programs. Understanding how to seek help and advocate for oneself or others is a crucial skill for beneficiaries, caregivers, and healthcare providers. Let's explore ways to effectively seek assistance and engage in advocacy.

Seeking Assistance with Medicaid and Medicare

- **State Health Insurance Assistance Programs (SHIP):** These programs offer free one-on-one counseling and assistance for Medicare beneficiaries. They can help with understanding coverage, enrollment, billing issues, and more.

- **Medicaid Offices:** Each state has a Medicaid office that can provide information and assistance regarding eligibility, coverage, and how to apply.

- **Online Resources:** Websites like Medicare.gov and Medicaid.gov offer comprehensive information and tools to manage benefits and find providers.

Advocating for Rights and Services

- **Understand Your Rights:** Beneficiaries should be aware of their rights under Medicaid and Medicare, including the right to appeal decisions and the right to receive necessary and appropriate healthcare services.

- **Effective Communication:** Clearly communicating with healthcare providers, insurance representatives, and program administrators is key to resolving issues and getting needed information.

- **Documenting Interactions:** Keep detailed records of all interactions, including dates, names, and summaries of conversations, when dealing with Medicaid, Medicare, or healthcare providers.

Utilizing Community Resources

- **Non-Profit Organizations:** Many non-profit organizations offer support and advocacy services for older adults and people with disabilities.

- **Legal Aid Services:** Free or low-cost legal services can help with understanding rights, appealing denials, and addressing other legal aspects of healthcare coverage.

Engaging in Policy Advocacy

- **Stay Informed:** Keep up-to-date with potential policy changes and understand how they might impact Medicaid and Medicare beneficiaries.

- **Join Advocacy Groups:** Participate in advocacy groups that work to protect and expand the rights and services of Medicaid and Medicare beneficiaries.

- **Contact Legislators:** Reach out to local and national legislators to express concerns and opinions about healthcare policies.

For Caregivers and Advocates

- **Educate Yourself:** Caregivers and advocates should educate themselves about the specifics of Medicaid and Medicare, including the latest changes and available services.

- **Networking:** Building relationships with healthcare providers, social workers, and other caregivers can provide additional support and resources.

Advocacy and seeking assistance are essential for effectively navigating Medicaid and Medicare. By utilizing available resources, understanding rights, and communicating effectively, beneficiaries can ensure they receive the care and services they are entitled to. Additionally, engaging in broader advocacy efforts can help shape policies for more equitable and accessible healthcare.

15.4. Exercise: 10 MCQs with Answers at the End

Test your understanding of the challenges, assistance, and advocacy related to Medicaid and Medicare. This exercise aims to assess your knowledge of navigating these programs, addressing common issues, and utilizing available resources.

1. **For assistance with Medicare-related issues, beneficiaries can contact:**

  A. State Health Insurance Assistance Programs (SHIP)

B. The Federal Trade Commission

C. Their local supermarket

D. Any online forum

2. One common challenge for Medicare and Medicaid beneficiaries is:

A. Too frequent policy changes

B. Understanding complex program rules

C. Mandatory volunteering for community services

D. Limited online resources

3. A valuable resource for understanding Medicaid coverage is:

A. The local gym

B. State Medicaid offices

C. Fashion magazines

D. Social media influencers

4. Effective advocacy for healthcare rights includes:

A. Ignoring policy changes

B. Documenting interactions and communications

C. Only relying on friends' advice

D. Refusing to contact healthcare providers

5. **The role of non-profit organizations in healthcare can involve:**

A. Providing entertainment services

B. Offering support and advocacy for beneficiaries

C. Selling health insurance

D. Providing legal representation in all cases

6. **To appeal a decision made by Medicare, beneficiaries should:**

A. Start a social media campaign

B. Contact a celebrity for support

C. Utilize the appeals process outlined by Medicare

D. Immediately give up on receiving services

7. **Medicaid and Medicare policy updates can be found on:**

A. Medicare.gov and Medicaid.gov

B. Any random website

C. Only in printed newspapers

D. Television soap operas

8. **Caregivers and advocates for beneficiaries should:**

A. Avoid learning about the healthcare system

B. Educate themselves about Medicaid and Medicare specifics

C. Refuse to communicate with medical professionals

D. Only rely on hearsay for information

9. **When facing challenges in Medicaid and Medicare, beneficiaries can seek help from:**

A. Legal aid services

B. Fast food restaurants

C. Fictional characters

D. Celebrity talk shows

10. **In advocating for policy changes in healthcare, individuals can:**

A. Only complain to friends

B. Contact local and national legislators

C. Refuse to learn about current policies

D. Avoid all forms of communication

Answers:

1. A. State Health Insurance Assistance Programs (SHIP)

2. B. Understanding complex program rules

3. B. State Medicaid offices

4. B. Documenting interactions and communications

5. B. Offering support and advocacy for beneficiaries

6. C. Utilize the appeals process outlined by Medicare

7. A. Medicare.gov and Medicaid.gov

8. B. Educate themselves about Medicaid and Medicare specifics

9. A. Legal aid services

10. B. Contact local and national legislators

These questions are designed to enhance your understanding of how to navigate the challenges and complexities of Medicaid and Medicare, and the importance of advocacy and seeking the right assistance.

Conclusion

As we conclude this comprehensive guide on Medicaid and Medicare, it's clear that navigating these programs involves understanding a broad spectrum of topics, from the basics of eligibility and coverage to more complex issues like policy changes, long-term care planning, and the integration of technology.

Key takeaways include:

- **Understanding Eligibility and Coverage:** Grasping the differences between Medicaid and Medicare, as well as the specific coverage and eligibility requirements of each program, is fundamental.

- **Staying Informed:** Keeping up-to-date with policy changes and leveraging resources like SHIP and state Medicaid offices can help beneficiaries make informed decisions.

- **Addressing Challenges:** Recognizing and addressing common challenges, such as program complexity and coverage gaps, is crucial for effective healthcare management.

- **Advocacy and Assistance:** Engaging in advocacy and seeking appropriate assistance are essential for maximizing benefits and navigating the healthcare system effectively.

- **Embracing Technology:** Understanding the evolving role of technology in healthcare, particularly in areas like telemedicine and e-health, can enhance healthcare delivery and accessibility.

- **Planning for the Future:** Preparing for future healthcare needs, including long-term care and end-of-life decisions, requires thoughtful consideration and planning.

This guide aims to provide a comprehensive overview, empowering beneficiaries, caregivers, and healthcare professionals to effectively navigate Medicaid and Medicare. By staying informed and proactive, individuals can ensure they receive the healthcare services they need while adapting to the ever-evolving landscape of these vital healthcare programs.

The best way to thank an author is to write a review.

www.ingramcontent.com/pod-product-compliance
Lightning Source LLC
LaVergne TN
LVHW010326200726
843507LV00010B/1377